The Power of Castor Oil

Complete Guide to Natural Remedies: 150+ Recipes for Radiant Skin Hair Growth and Overall Wellness

OptiLife Publishing

"Nature itself is the best physician" — Hippocrates

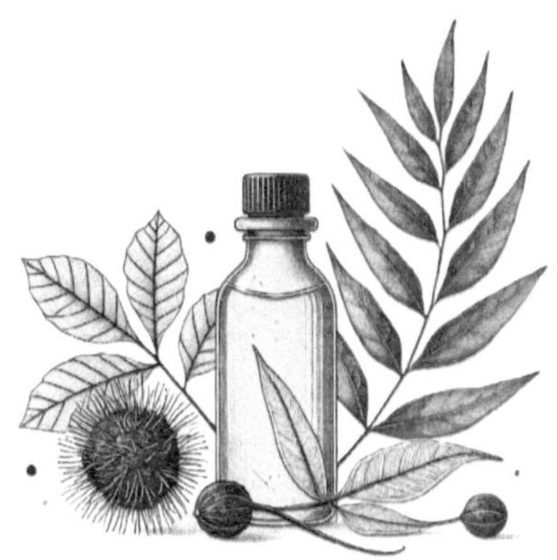

About the author

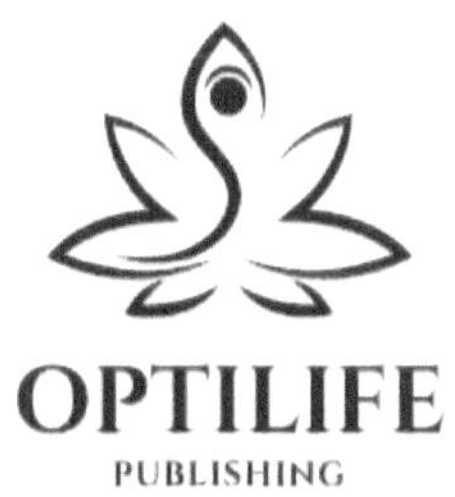

Optilife Publishing is at the forefront of the wellness revolution, dedicated to empowering individuals with cutting-edge knowledge and tools for optimal living. We specialize in curating and delivering high-quality, insightful books that explore the transformative power of holistic and alternative medicine, biohacking, and groundbreaking health strategies.

Our mission is to bridge the gap between ancient wisdom and modern science, offering readers practical, evidence-based solutions for enhancing mind, body, and spirit. From the powerful potentials of psilocybin microdosing and cognitive behavioral therapy (CBT) to the life-changing possibilities of hypnosis, peptides, and beyond, Optilife Publishing is your trusted guide on the journey to optimal health and well-being.

As we continue to expand our library, our focus remains on exploring the uncharted territories of human potential, bringing innovative approaches to health and wellness that are both effective and accessible. Whether you're seeking to unlock your mind's potential, rejuvenate your body, or enhance your overall quality of life, Optilife Publishing provides the knowledge you need to live your best life.

Join us on this journey to discover the future of wellness, one book at a time.

Contents

Introduction

At OptiLife, we've always believed in the power of nature to heal, but it wasn't until our CEO, Sarah, faced a personal struggle that castor oil became a core part of our philosophy. Sarah had battled thinning hair for years. No matter how many pricey serums or treatments she tried, nothing seemed to work. It was frustrating, more than frustrating, it was a blow to her confidence. Hair isn't just about beauty; it's about feeling good in your own skin, and when it starts thinning, it can feel like you're losing a part of yourself.

One day, in a casual office conversation, a colleague mentioned castor oil. Sarah wasn't convinced, how could a simple oil from a seed do what high-end products couldn't? But at that point, she had nothing to lose. So she started applying it, skeptically at first. Slowly but surely, her hair started to regain its health. It wasn't an overnight transformation, but after a few months, the results were undeniable thicker, shinier hair that felt vibrant again. And with that, our journey into the world of castor oil began.

The Struggles We All Face

Like many of us, Sarah's story is one of frustration with the overwhelming number of products and promises that just don't seem to work. Dry skin, thinning hair, irritated scalps, these are problems that millions of people face every day. And yet, the beauty industry often offers solutions that are expensive, filled with synthetic ingredients, and ultimately underwhelming.

We've been there too, which is why this book exists. We wanted to create a resource that offers something different, a natural, effective alternative that's easy to incorporate into your life. Castor oil has been quietly delivering results for centuries, and it's time to rediscover its benefits.

Castor Oil: A Natural Solution with a Long Legacy

Castor oil isn't new. In fact, it's been used for thousands of years across various cultures, from ancient Egypt to modern holistic practices. Its appeal is simple: it's versatile, natural, and deeply nourishing. Whether you're looking to hydrate dry skin, support healthy hair growth, or soothe irritated areas, castor oil offers a gentle, natural way to enhance your beauty and wellness routines.

The key lies in its rich fatty acid content, particularly ricinoleic acid, which works to deeply moisturize and support the skin's natural barrier while promoting healthier hair. Castor oil isn't a quick fix, but when used consistently, it can become a cornerstone of your daily self-care.

Our Commitment to Natural Wellness

At OptiLife, we're passionate about finding real, sustainable solutions for everyday problems. Sarah's personal experience with castor oil wasn't just a turning point for her, it inspired all of us to explore how this oil could help others. We've spent years researching, testing, and perfecting ways to use castor oil, and now, we're excited to share what we've learned with you.

This book is designed to be more than just a list of recipes. It's a guide that will help you understand how to make the most of castor oil in your life. We believe in practical solutions, and this book will give you the tools to create effective, natural treatments for your skin, hair, and wellness needs.

What You Can Expect from This Book

Inside these pages, you'll find everything you need to know about using castor oil to support your beauty and wellness. We start by exploring the rich history and scientific foundations of castor oil, so you can understand why it has been trusted for centuries. From ancient uses to modern scientific research, we cover how castor oil works and why it's so effective.

The heart of this book, however, lies in the 150 recipes we've developed. These recipes are designed to be simple, effective, and easy to follow. Whether you're looking for a soothing face serum, a hair mask to encourage growth, or a natural remedy for dry skin, you'll find a variety of options tailored to different needs. Each recipe comes with clear, step-by-step instructions, so even if you're new to DIY treatments, you'll be able to follow along with ease.

Beyond the recipes, we've also included practical tips on how to make castor oil work for you. We'll show you how to customize treatments to suit your specific needs and guide you through the process of integrating these solutions into your daily routine. The goal is to empower you to take control of your wellness in a way that feels manageable and sustainable.

The Science Behind Castor Oil

While castor oil has been used for centuries, modern science has given us a deeper understanding of why it works so well. The secret lies in ricinoleic acid, a unique fatty acid that has anti-inflammatory and moisturizing properties. This acid helps to soothe irritated skin, support healthy hair growth, and keep the skin's natural barrier strong and hydrated.

Studies have shown that castor oil can improve skin hydration, reduce inflammation, and even encourage hair growth by improving circulation to the scalp. It's a natural solution that works in harmony with your body's own processes, offering gentle yet effective support for your everyday health and beauty needs.

Ready to Try It for Yourself?

We know that trying something new can feel intimidating, especially if you've been disappointed by products in the past. But castor oil is different. It's a simple, affordable option that's easy to incorporate into your routine, whether you're looking to solve a specific issue or just enhance your overall wellness.

This book is here to guide you through that process. With 150 recipes, you'll have a wealth of options to explore, from skincare and haircare to wellness and even household uses. Each recipe has been carefully crafted to help you get the most out of castor oil, no matter what your goals are.

Start Your Journey Today

We wrote this book because we believe in the power of small, consistent changes. Castor oil may seem like a humble product, but when used regularly, it can make a big difference in how you feel about your skin, your hair, and your health. You don't need to make a dramatic shift overnight, just start with one recipe, see how it works for you, and go from there.

Your journey with castor oil starts here. Whether you're looking to boost your beauty routine or find natural solutions for everyday wellness, this book will help you discover the many benefits of this versatile, time-tested oil. Welcome to a new chapter of natural care, where simplicity meets effectiveness, and nature offers the solutions we need.

Chapter One

Unveiling the Secrets of Castor Oil

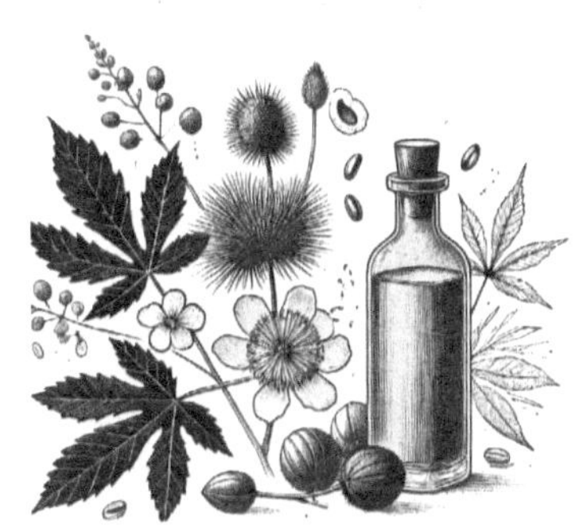

C astor oil is one of nature's most versatile and enduring remedies. Its use spans thousands of years, crossing continents and cultures, and its applications range from beauty rituals to medicinal treatments. In this chapter, we'll explore the fascinating history of castor oil, uncovering how it became a staple in ancient civilizations and continues to be valued in modern wellness practices. From ancient Egyptian beauty secrets to Ayurvedic healing, castor oil has left an indelible mark on history.

The Ancient Legacy of Castor Oil

To understand why castor oil has persisted for thousands of years, we need to dive into its origins and significance across various civilizations. Long before modern science validated its benefits, people from different cultures recognized its powerful properties and incorporated it into their daily lives for a variety of purposes.

Historical Significance Across Civilizations

Castor oil's journey begins in ancient times, where it played a crucial role in the health, beauty, and religious practices of early societies. It was prized for its ability to heal, nourish, and preserve, making it an indispensable part of everyday life.

Castor oil has been found in early texts and archaeological findings, indicating its widespread use from Africa to Asia and the Mediterranean. Its early adoption by various cultures speaks volumes about its perceived value, even in times when little was understood about its actual chemical properties.

From early civilizations, the oil was used in lamps, as a beauty aid, and for its healing properties. However, it wasn't just its practical benefits that made castor oil popular, it held spiritual and cultural significance as well. The reverence ancient peoples had for castor oil suggests they understood its power not just as a remedy but as something almost sacred.

Ancient Egyptian Medicine: The Beauty Elixir of the Pharaohs

In ancient Egypt, castor oil was considered a highly prized commodity. Cleopatra, one of history's most iconic figures, is often associated with beauty secrets that have endured for centuries. Among these, castor oil stood out for its moisturizing properties and its role in keeping skin soft and smooth in the harsh desert climate.

Beyond beauty, the Egyptians also used castor oil medicinally. Physicians of the time would prescribe it as a natural remedy for digestive issues and skin problems. It was applied to wounds, used to soothe inflammation, and even employed as a laxative. Castor oil's versatility made it a must-have for anyone seeking to maintain health and vitality.

The oil was so revered that it was often found in the tombs of pharaohs. Archaeologists have discovered small vials of castor oil placed carefully alongside the deceased, a testament to its perceived value in both life and the afterlife. This practice underscores the idea that castor oil wasn't just a daily necessity, it was a symbol of well-being and care that transcended death.

One of the most important documents in medical history, the **Ebers Papyrus**, also references castor oil. This ancient text, dating back to around 1550 BC, is one of the earliest medical documents we have and includes recipes for treating a variety of ailments, many of which call for castor oil. Its inclusion in such a foundational text underscores its importance in Egyptian medicine.

Ayurvedic Practices in India: Healing from the Inside Out

While castor oil was revered in Egypt for its external benefits, in India, it became a cornerstone of **Ayurveda**, one of the world's oldest holistic healing systems. Ayurveda, which translates to "the science of life," emphasizes the balance between mind, body, and spirit, and castor oil plays a crucial role in maintaining this balance.

In Ayurvedic practice, castor oil is used both internally and externally to promote overall health. Internally, it is often used as a mild laxative to cleanse the body of toxins. According to Ayurveda, the buildup of toxins can disrupt the body's natural balance, leading to illness. Castor oil's purgative properties help to flush out these toxins, supporting digestive health and maintaining internal harmony.

Externally, castor oil is used to treat skin disorders, alleviate joint pain, and reduce inflammation. It is applied in **Abhyanga**, a traditional Ayurvedic massage, where warm castor oil is massaged into the skin to enhance circulation, nourish tissues, and calm the nervous system. This practice not only promotes physical health but is also believed to foster mental clarity and emotional balance.

In Ayurveda, castor oil is also known for its ability to balance **Vata** and **Kapha** doshas, two of the body's primary energies that govern physiological and psychological functions. Vata, associated with movement and air, can lead to dryness and stiffness when out of balance, while Kapha, associated with water and earth, can cause lethargy and congestion. Castor oil helps by grounding Vata and clearing excess Kapha, making it a valuable remedy in maintaining overall equilibrium.

Roman and Greek Therapeutic Uses: The Oil of Healing

As castor oil traveled westward, it became a key player in the health practices of the **Roman** and **Greek** empires. Both cultures were known for their advancements in medicine and valued castor oil for its medicinal properties. Physicians of the time, including Hippocrates, often prescribed castor oil for its ability to treat various ailments, particularly digestive and skin conditions.

In **Roman** culture, castor oil was commonly used as a laxative, a practice that continues in some parts of the world today. The Greeks, like the Egyptians, also valued it for its ability to soothe skin conditions and reduce inflammation. Castor oil was often applied to wounds to speed up healing and to alleviate pain associated with sore muscles and joints.

Greek texts from this period reference castor oil as a treatment for eye conditions, particularly for reducing irritation and swelling. Its use in ancient Greece shows that castor oil was recognized not just for its external applications but also for its ability to soothe internal discomforts. The widespread use of castor oil in these advanced societies further cemented its reputation as a reliable natural remedy.

Cultural Relevance: A Sacred Oil Across Rituals and Ceremonies

Throughout history, castor oil has been more than just a medicinal or cosmetic product, it has been a symbol of purity, healing, and protection. In many ancient cultures, castor oil was used in rituals and ceremonies, often believed to carry spiritual significance.

In ancient Egypt, it was used in burial rites, placed in tombs to accompany the dead into the afterlife. It was thought to provide sustenance and care for the soul's journey beyond the physical world. This speaks to the reverence Egyptians had for castor oil, not just as a practical remedy but as a sacred element in their spiritual practices.

In **India**, castor oil was (and still is) used in **religious ceremonies**. It is often applied to idols in Hindu temples as a symbol of purification and protection. The oil's ability to cleanse, nourish, and protect made it a fitting choice for use in rituals intended to honor deities and invite blessings. Castor oil lamps, known as **Diyas**, are still lit during festivals like **Diwali**, symbolizing the dispelling of darkness and ignorance with the light of knowledge and purity.

The oil's role in such rituals emphasizes its deeper cultural relevance. It wasn't just used for health and beauty, it was a powerful symbol of healing, protection, and connection to the divine.

Medicinal Uses in Traditional Chinese Medicine

Across the globe in ancient **China**, castor oil became a key element in **Traditional Chinese Medicine (TCM)**. Castor oil, known as **"Bi Ma You"** in Chinese, was recognized for its ability to clear heat and remove toxins from the body. In TCM, castor oil was often applied externally to treat skin conditions such as boils, abscesses, and other inflammatory skin disorders.

In addition to treating external ailments, Chinese herbalists used castor oil to alleviate internal imbalances. Like in Ayurvedic practices, it was sometimes taken as a laxative to remove heat from the intestines and promote digestive health. Castor oil was also used to soothe joint pain and arthritis, with practitioners often combining it with other medicinal herbs to enhance its effects.

The incorporation of castor oil into TCM speaks to its adaptability across different healing systems. While each culture approached medicine differently, castor oil's consistent presence across them shows its undeniable effectiveness in promoting health and wellness.

Documentation and Artifacts: Castor Oil's Lasting Imprint on History

The evidence of castor oil's historical use is not only found in texts but also in the physical artifacts and remains left behind. As mentioned earlier, castor oil has been discovered in the tombs of ancient Egyptians, preserved in jars alongside the bodies of the deceased. These finds have provided us with concrete proof of castor oil's importance in ancient life.

The **Ebers Papyrus**, one of the oldest known medical texts, dating back to 1550 BC, contains dozens of remedies that call for castor oil. This document is a treasure trove of medical knowledge from ancient Egypt and demonstrates how integral castor oil was in the treatment of ailments ranging from eye irritations to digestive issues.

In **India**, ancient Ayurvedic texts reference castor oil as a key ingredient in various medicinal treatments, further underscoring its role in holistic healing. These texts, still studied and followed today, provide a bridge between the ancient and modern uses of castor oil, showing that its value has endured through millennia.

Ebers Papyrus References: A Window into Ancient Medicine

The **Ebers Papyrus** is an essential piece of historical evidence that underscores the importance of castor oil in ancient medical practices. This ancient Egyptian document, discovered in the 19th century, is one of the earliest and most comprehensive medical texts known to exist. It outlines treatments for a wide array of conditions, many of which include the use of castor oil.

The fact that castor oil is mentioned so frequently in the **Ebers Papyrus** speaks to its widespread use and efficacy. Even today, many of the treatments listed in the papyrus are being revisited by modern herbalists and natural medicine practitioners, continuing the legacy of this powerful oil.

Discoveries in Egyptian Tombs: Castor Oil's Enduring Value

One of the most fascinating aspects of castor oil's history is its presence in Egyptian tombs. The discovery of small vials of castor oil in the burial chambers of pharaohs highlights its significance as a valued resource in both life and death. Egyptians believed that the items placed in tombs were essential for the afterlife, meaning that castor oil wasn't just seen as a product for earthly existence, but as something valuable beyond death.

The tombs of prominent figures, including **King Tutankhamun**, contained evidence of castor oil, further reinforcing the notion that it was a luxury reserved for the elite. Its inclusion in such important burials illustrates the reverence Egyptians had for the oil and its potential to provide comfort and healing, not just in this life, but in the journey that followed.

Enduring Legacy: The Timeless Appeal of Castor Oil

Despite the advancements in modern medicine, castor oil remains a valuable and respected remedy. Its endurance across civilizations is a testament to its versatility and effectiveness. While ancient cultures may not have had the scientific tools to understand why castor oil worked, they knew from experience that it did.

Today, castor oil continues to be a go-to solution for those seeking natural, gentle remedies. It is widely used in modern Ayurveda, naturopathy, and even in beauty products that emphasize organic, sustainable ingredients. From its role in ancient Egyptian beauty rituals to its current popularity in DIY skincare and haircare, castor oil's legacy is one of simplicity, effectiveness, and timelessness.

As we continue to uncover more about the benefits of castor oil, both through historical evidence and modern research, one thing remains clear: castor oil has stood the test of time for a reason. Its rich history and enduring use are a testament to its remarkable versatility and its ability to provide gentle, natural care that has been cherished for millennia.

Key Takeaway: Castor oil's journey through history, from the tombs of ancient Egypt to modern holistic health practices, reveals a product that has been cherished for its healing properties for thousands of years. Whether used for beauty, medicine, or spiritual rituals, castor oil's legacy continues to thrive, offering us a natural, time-tested solution that endures through generations.

Chapter Two

The Science Behind Castor Oil's Potency

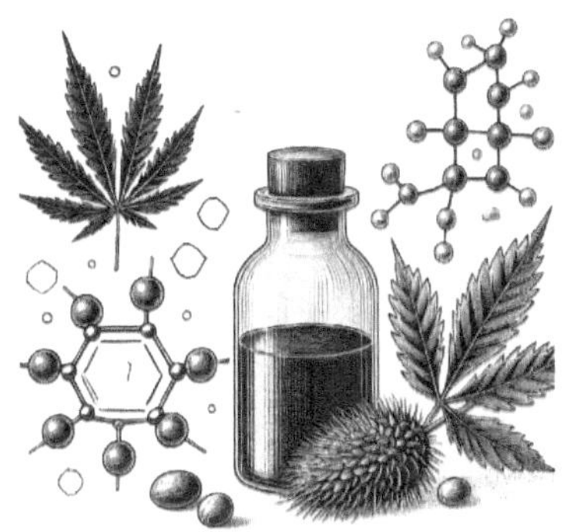

Castor oil is not just an ancient remedy with historical significance; it's also backed by modern science. Understanding its chemical composition and how it interacts with the body sheds light on why it has remained such a powerful natural solution for so many different health and beauty applications. In this chapter, we will dive into the science behind castor oil's potency, exploring its unique chemical properties, how it works within the body, and the studies that support its effectiveness.

Chemical Composition: The Building Blocks of Potency

At first glance, castor oil may seem like a simple substance. It's a thick, pale yellow oil extracted from the seeds of the **Ricinus communis** plant, also known as the castor bean plant. But what makes castor oil stand out among other natural oils is its unique chemical composition, which is responsible for its wide range of benefits.

High Ricinoleic Acid Content: The Secret Ingredient

The primary component of castor oil is **ricinoleic acid**, a monounsaturated fatty acid that accounts for about 85-90% of the oil's composition. Ricinoleic acid is what sets castor oil apart from other plant-based oils. This fatty acid has unique properties that give castor oil its potent moisturizing, anti-inflammatory, and healing capabilities.

Ricinoleic acid is known for its ability to penetrate deeply into the skin, providing intense hydration. Unlike many oils that simply sit on the skin's surface, ricinoleic acid absorbs into the layers of the skin, creating a protective barrier that locks in moisture. This deep-penetrating action is why castor oil is often used in treatments for dry, cracked skin and to restore moisture to damaged hair.

But ricinoleic acid doesn't just hydrate, it also has anti-inflammatory properties. Studies have shown that it can reduce swelling and inflammation when applied topically. This makes castor oil an effective remedy for conditions like eczema, psoriasis, and even joint pain. Its anti-inflammatory action is one of the reasons it has been used for centuries in both beauty and medicinal practices.

Omega-9 Fatty Acids: Nourishment for Skin and Hair

In addition to its high ricinoleic acid content, castor oil also contains **omega-9 fatty acids**, which are essential for maintaining healthy skin and hair. Omega-9s, also known as oleic acid, help to nourish and strengthen the skin's natural barrier, protecting it from environmental damage and promoting a youthful, healthy appearance.

These fatty acids also play a key role in improving hair health. Omega-9s are known to strengthen hair follicles, reduce breakage, and promote smoother, shinier hair. For individuals dealing with dry, brittle hair or scalp conditions, the omega-9 fatty acids in castor oil provide much-needed moisture and protection. Combined with ricinoleic acid, omega-9 fatty acids contribute to castor oil's overall effectiveness in treating a wide range of skin and hair concerns.

Mechanism of Action: How Castor Oil Works

Understanding how castor oil works within the body and on the skin gives us insight into why it's so effective. While the oil's composition is important, the way it interacts with biological systems is what allows it to deliver its benefits.

Anti-inflammatory Pathways: Soothing from the Inside Out

One of the key ways that castor oil works is through its **anti-inflammatory pathways**. Ricinoleic acid, the primary component of castor oil, has been shown to activate receptors in the skin and body that reduce inflammation. These receptors, known as **EP3 prostanoid receptors**, are part of the body's natural anti-inflammatory response system.

When castor oil is applied to inflamed or irritated skin, ricinoleic acid interacts with these receptors, reducing the release of inflammatory compounds like prostaglandins. This helps to soothe the skin, reduce redness, and calm conditions such as dermatitis, rosacea, and eczema. The anti-inflammatory properties of ricinoleic acid also make castor oil effective for reducing pain in conditions like arthritis and sore muscles, where inflammation plays a major role.

This mechanism of action is one of the reasons why castor oil has been used for so long in both traditional and modern medicine. Whether it's applied to aching joints or irritated skin, the oil's ability to interact with the body's natural anti-inflammatory pathways allows it to provide relief in a way that few other natural remedies can.

Moisturizing Properties: Locking in Hydration

In addition to its anti-inflammatory effects, castor oil's powerful moisturizing properties are a key part of how it works. The oil forms a protective layer on the skin, preventing moisture from escaping. This is especially important for individuals with dry or damaged skin, as it helps to restore the skin's natural hydration balance.

Castor oil's ability to deeply penetrate the skin makes it a superior moisturizer. Many commercial moisturizers only sit on the surface of the skin, providing temporary relief. Castor oil, on the other hand, works from within, hydrating the deeper layers of the skin and creating long-lasting moisture retention. This is why it's often used in treatments for severely dry skin, chapped lips, and cracked heels.

The same moisturizing properties apply to hair. When castor oil is massaged into the scalp and hair, it helps to nourish and strengthen the hair shaft, reducing breakage and improving overall hair texture. The oil's thick consistency allows it to coat the hair strands, sealing in moisture and preventing damage from heat, chemicals, and environmental factors.

Clinical Studies and Research: The Science Behind the Benefits

Over the years, a growing body of research has emerged to support the traditional uses of castor oil. While ancient cultures relied on anecdotal evidence and experience, modern science has provided us with a deeper understanding of why castor oil works so well for skin, hair, and health.

Studies on Skin Hydration: A Natural Moisturizer

Several studies highlight the moisturizing benefits of castor oil, primarily due to its high ricinoleic acid content. Research from sources like **Skin Type Solutions** and the **Journal of Cosmetic Science** emphasizes that ricinoleic acid helps create an occlusive barrier on the skin, locking in moisture and reducing transepidermal water loss (TEWL). This is particularly beneficial for dry or irritated skin, as the oil deeply penetrates the layers of the skin to provide long-lasting hydration. The fatty acids in castor oil act as humectants, which attract moisture to the skin, making it an excellent choice for individuals with dry or dehydrated skin (Int J Naturopath Med)(Skin Type Solutions) .

The study also noted that castor oil's thick, viscous texture allowed it to create a more substantial barrier on the skin than lighter oils like coconut or olive oil. This barrier effect is crucial for individuals living in dry or cold climates, where the skin is more prone to moisture loss. Castor oil's ability to lock in hydration and protect the skin from environmental stressors makes it a superior natural moisturizer.

Research on Hair Growth Stimulation: Supporting Healthy Hair

While specific large-scale clinical studies on castor oil for hair growth are limited, there is research to support the idea that ricinoleic acid can stimulate circulation and prostaglandin production, which may promote hair growth. **The International Journal of Trichology** mentions that castor oil's high concentration of ricinoleic acid helps increase blood flow to the scalp, nourishing hair follicles and potentially leading to thicker, healthier hair (Pretty farm girl)(Skin Type Solutions). Furthermore, castor oil has been known for its ability to strengthen hair and prevent breakage, making it popular in hair care routines aimed at improving hair density.

Incorporating castor oil into a consistent routine, especially when massaged into the scalp, could provide cumulative benefits for hair health and growth, although more research is needed to conclusively prove this (My Blog).

These studies provide scientific backing for the long-held belief that castor oil is an effective remedy for hair loss and damaged hair. By increasing blood flow and stimulating hair follicles, castor oil supports healthier, fuller hair without the need for harsh chemicals or expensive treatments.

Understanding the Chemical Composition: A Detailed Breakdown

While we've already touched on the key components of castor oil, a more detailed breakdown of its chemical composition helps to clarify why it's so effective in various applications.

Detailed Breakdown: The Key Components

- **Ricinoleic Acid**: As mentioned, ricinoleic acid is the star of castor oil's composition, making up about 85-90% of the oil. It provides most of the oil's moisturizing, anti-inflammatory, and antimicrobial properties.

- **Oleic Acid (Omega-9 Fatty Acid)**: This fatty acid helps to nourish the skin and hair, strengthening the skin's barrier and promoting elasticity in the hair.

- **Linoleic Acid (Omega-6 Fatty Acid)**: Linoleic acid is an essential fatty acid that helps to soothe irritated skin and regulate moisture levels.

- **Vitamin E**: Castor oil also contains small amounts of **vitamin E**, a powerful antioxidant that protects the skin and hair from damage caused by free radicals and environmental stressors.

Comparative Analysis with Other Oils

When comparing castor oil to other popular natural oils like coconut, olive, or jojoba oil, its unique chemical makeup becomes even more apparent. While oils like coconut and jojoba are known for their light texture and rapid absorption, castor oil's thick consistency allows it to penetrate deeper into the skin and hair, providing longer-lasting hydration.

In terms of hair care, castor oil has a more robust ability to coat and protect hair strands than lighter oils like olive or argan oil. This makes it ideal for individuals with coarse or thick hair that needs extra moisture. Castor oil's ability to stimulate hair growth also sets it apart from other oils, making it a popular choice for individuals dealing with hair thinning or slow hair growth.

Impacts on Skin and Hair: Nourishment from the Inside Out

The combination of fatty acids, antioxidants, and anti-inflammatory compounds in castor oil makes it a powerful solution for both skin and hair health. When applied to the skin, castor oil penetrates deep into the layers of the dermis, providing hydration and reducing irritation from within. This makes it effective for treating dry patches, eczema, and even acne, as its antimicrobial properties help to reduce the bacteria that can cause breakouts.

For hair, castor oil nourishes the scalp, improves blood circulation, and strengthens hair follicles. This not only promotes hair growth but also reduces breakage and split ends, leading to healthier, shinier hair.

Potential Allergens: Safe Use and Precautions

While castor oil is generally considered safe for most people, it's important to be aware of potential allergens and sensitivities. Some individuals may experience skin irritation or allergic reactions when using castor oil, especially if they have sensitive skin. It's always recommended to perform a patch test before applying castor oil to larger areas of the skin or scalp.

If you experience any redness, itching, or swelling after using castor oil, it's best to discontinue use and consult with a healthcare professional. Allergic reactions to castor oil are rare, but they can occur in sensitive individuals.

For those considering taking castor oil internally, it's essential to follow dosage recommendations carefully. While castor oil has been used as a laxative for centuries, overuse can lead to digestive issues or dehydration. As with any natural remedy, moderation is key to safe and effective use.

Key Takeaway: The science behind castor oil's potency lies in its unique chemical composition, particularly its high ricinoleic acid content. This fatty acid gives castor oil its powerful moisturizing, anti-inflammatory, and healing properties, making it a versatile and effective solution for skin, hair, and overall wellness. With a growing body of research supporting its benefits, castor oil continues to be a valuable natural remedy for a wide range of health and beauty concerns.

Recipe Categories

In this section, we dive into the heart of the book: practical and effective recipes that allow you to harness the full potential of castor oil for skincare. From anti-aging treatments to personalized serums for different skin types, these recipes are designed to fit seamlessly into your daily routine and address a range of common skin concerns. Let's explore each category and how castor oil's unique properties work to nourish, hydrate, and protect the skin.

Chapter Three

Skincare (40 Recipes)

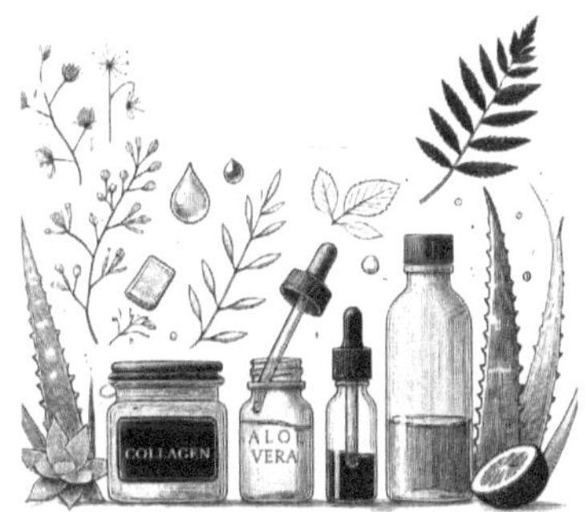

Anti-Aging with Castor Oil

Aging is a natural part of life, but that doesn't mean we can't support our skin as it changes. Castor oil is rich in ricinoleic acid and fatty acids that deeply penetrate the skin to promote hydration and improve elasticity. These properties make it an excellent choice for anti-aging treatments aimed at reducing fine lines, wrinkles, and sagging skin.

1. Castor Oil & Rosehip Anti-Wrinkle Night Serum

This night serum is designed for deep hydration and wrinkle reduction. The combination of castor oil and rosehip oil brings together two powerful anti-aging ingredients. Castor oil's ricinoleic acid penetrates the skin, locking in moisture, while rosehip oil is rich in vitamins A and C, which promote collagen production and skin regeneration.

Ingredients:

1 tablespoon castor oil

1 teaspoon rosehip oil

2 vitamin E capsules (pierced for the oil)

Instructions:

- Mix the castor oil, rosehip oil, and vitamin E oil in a small glass bottle with a dropper.

- After cleansing your face at night, apply 2-3 drops of the serum to your fingertips.

- Gently pat the serum onto your face, starting at your cheeks and working your way out to your forehead and chin. Be sure to focus on areas with wrinkles, such as around the eyes and mouth.

- Use upward, circular motions to massage the serum into your skin, allowing the oils to absorb fully. The upward motion helps fight the effects of gravity on the skin's firmness.

- Leave it on overnight to allow your skin to absorb the nutrients and hydrate deeply while you sleep.

2. Castor Oil & Aloe Vera Hydrating Mask

This hydrating mask soothes and nourishes dry, tired skin. Aloe vera provides a cooling, calming effect, while honey is a natural humectant that draws moisture into the skin. Combined with castor oil, this mask provides deep hydration and helps restore the skin's natural glow.

Ingredients:

1 tablespoon castor oil

2 tablespoons fresh aloe vera gel

1 teaspoon honey

Instructions:

- In a clean bowl, mix together the castor oil, fresh aloe vera gel, and honey until you get a smooth consistency.

- Start with a clean, dry face. Using your fingertips or a brush, evenly apply the mask to your entire face, avoiding the eye area.

- Gently massage the mask into your skin using small, circular motions. This helps increase blood circulation and ensures that the ingredients penetrate deeper.

- Let the mask sit for 20 minutes. During this time, the aloe vera will soothe your skin while the castor oil hydrates.

- After 20 minutes, rinse your face with lukewarm water, using a soft cloth to gently remove any remaining mask.

- Pat your face dry with a clean towel and follow up with a lightweight moisturizer to lock in hydration.

3. Castor Oil & Frankincense Firming Serum

Frankincense oil is well-known for its skin-tightening properties. In this serum, it works alongside castor oil to firm the skin and reduce fine lines. Regular use of this serum helps improve skin elasticity and can leave your skin feeling tighter and more youthful.

Ingredients:

1 tablespoon castor oil

1 teaspoon jojoba oil

5 drops frankincense essential oil

Instructions:

- In a small bottle, combine the castor oil, jojoba oil, and frankincense essential oil.

- Cleanse your face thoroughly before applying the serum. It's important to start with clean skin to ensure the serum penetrates deeply.

- Apply 2-3 drops of the serum to your fingertips and warm it between your hands by rubbing them together.

- Starting from your neck and working upward, gently massage the serum into your skin. Focus on areas that show signs of aging, such as your neck, jawline, and forehead.

- Massage in upward, circular motions for a few minutes to promote blood circulation and ensure deep absorption.

- Leave the serum on overnight and rinse your face in the morning if needed. Repeat this treatment nightly for the best results.

4. Castor Oil & Coffee Ground Exfoliating Scrub

This scrub combines the exfoliating power of coffee grounds with the nourishing properties of castor oil to remove dead skin cells and reveal fresh, glowing skin.

Ingredients:

2 tablespoons castor oil

1 tablespoon used coffee grounds

1 teaspoon coconut oil

Instructions:

- In a bowl, mix together the castor oil, used coffee grounds, and coconut oil.

- After washing your face with warm water to open your pores, gently apply the scrub to your damp skin.

- Use your fingertips to massage the scrub in small circular motions, concentrating on areas with dead skin buildup or dryness, such as the forehead, nose, and chin.

- Avoid scrubbing too harshly, especially around delicate areas like the eyes.

- After 2-3 minutes of exfoliation, rinse your face with lukewarm water until all of the scrub is removed.

- Pat your skin dry and follow up with a moisturizer to keep your skin hydrated and smooth.

5. Castor Oil & Pomegranate Antioxidant Serum

Pomegranate seed oil is packed with antioxidants that help neutralize free radicals, which contribute to premature aging. When combined with castor oil, this serum provides an antioxidant boost that can help protect the skin from environmental damage and encourage cell regeneration.

Ingredients:

1 tablespoon castor oil

1 tablespoon pomegranate seed oil

5 drops lavender essential oil

Instructions:

- Combine the castor oil, pomegranate seed oil, and lavender essential oil in a dropper bottle and shake gently to mix.

- Cleanse your face and pat dry.

- Apply 3-4 drops of the serum onto your fingers and rub them together to warm the oil.

- Gently press the serum into your skin, focusing on areas that are most exposed to environmental stress, such as your forehead, cheeks, and chin.

- Use upward, circular motions to massage the serum into your skin, ensuring it's evenly distributed.

- Allow the serum to fully absorb before applying your moisturizer or makeup.

- Use this serum every evening to protect and nourish your skin.

6. Castor Oil & Turmeric Brightening Mask

Turmeric is known for its anti-inflammatory and brightening properties, making this mask ideal for those looking to brighten dull skin and even out skin tone. Paired with castor oil, this mask provides moisture while also targeting dark spots and uneven pigmentation.

Ingredients:

1 tablespoon castor oil

1 teaspoon turmeric powder

1 tablespoon yogurt

Instructions:

- In a small bowl, mix the castor oil, turmeric powder, and yogurt until you get a smooth paste.

- After cleansing your face, apply the mask evenly using your fingertips or a brush, avoiding the eye area.

- Let the mask sit for 15 minutes to allow the turmeric to work its brightening magic.

- Rinse thoroughly with warm water, using a soft cloth to gently remove any remaining mask. Be mindful of turmeric's natural staining properties; use an old towel to dry your face.

- Follow up with a toner and lightweight moisturizer to lock in moisture.

- Use this mask once a week for best results.

7. Castor Oil & Avocado Rich Cream

This rich, nourishing cream is perfect for mature or dry skin. The combination of avocado oil and shea butter provides intense moisture while castor oil helps repair and rejuvenate the skin.

Ingredients:

1 tablespoon castor oil

1 tablespoon avocado oil

2 teaspoons shea butter

Instructions:

- Melt the shea butter in a double boiler over low heat until liquefied.

- Stir in the castor oil and avocado oil until well combined.

- Allow the mixture to cool at room temperature, then refrigerate until it starts to solidify.

- Whip the cream with a hand mixer until it becomes light and fluffy.

- Store the cream in a clean, airtight jar. Apply a small amount to your face and neck at night, massaging it into your skin with upward strokes.

- Let the cream absorb overnight for deep hydration and repair.

8. Castor Oil & Carrot Seed Oil Eye Treatment

Carrot seed oil is rich in antioxidants that promote cell regeneration, making it ideal for treating the delicate skin around the eyes. This treatment helps reduce puffiness, fine lines, and dark circles.

Ingredients:

1 tablespoon castor oil

1 teaspoon carrot seed oil

2 drops rose essential oil

Instructions:

- Mix the castor oil, carrot seed oil, and rose essential oil in a small dropper bottle.

- After cleansing your face, use your fingertip to apply a small amount of the oil to the area under your eyes.

- Gently tap the oil into your skin, taking care not to rub or pull on the delicate skin around the eyes.

- Allow the oil to absorb fully before going to bed. Use nightly for best results in reducing puffiness and fine lines.

9. Castor Oil & Grape Seed Oil Anti-Wrinkle Moisturizer

This lightweight moisturizer is perfect for daily use, with grape seed oil offering antioxidants that help protect against skin aging and rosemary oil providing an uplifting scent. Castor oil locks in moisture, making this a hydrating and protective solution.

Ingredients:

1 tablespoon castor oil

1 tablespoon grape seed oil

5 drops rosemary essential oil

Instructions:

- Mix the castor oil, grape seed oil, and rosemary essential oil in a small bottle.

- After cleansing your face in the morning, apply 3-4 drops of the moisturizer to your fingertips.

- Gently massage it into your face and neck, using upward strokes to promote circulation and prevent sagging.

- Let the moisturizer fully absorb before applying makeup or sunscreen.

- Use daily to keep your skin hydrated and protected from free radical damage, helping to reduce the appearance of fine lines and wrinkles.

10. Castor Oil & Hyaluronic Acid Hydration Boost

This serum combines the powerful hydrating properties of hyaluronic acid, which holds up to 1,000 times its weight in water, with castor oil's moisturizing effects. Together, they help plump the skin and reduce fine lines, making it a perfect solution for dehydrated skin.

Ingredients:

1 tablespoon castor oil

1 teaspoon hyaluronic acid serum

Instructions:

- Mix the castor oil and hyaluronic acid serum in a small dropper bottle.

- After cleansing your face, leave it slightly damp—hyaluronic acid works best on moist skin.

- Apply 2-3 drops of the serum to your fingertips and gently press it into your skin, focusing on dry or wrinkled areas.

- Use upward, circular motions to help the serum absorb into the deeper layers of your skin.

- Once the serum is fully absorbed, follow with a lightweight moisturizer to lock in hydration.

- Use this serum morning and night for maximum hydration and plumping effects.

11. Castor Oil & Vitamin C Brightening Serum

Vitamin C is a well-known antioxidant that helps brighten the skin and reduce hyperpigmentation. This serum combines vitamin C with castor oil, providing hydration while evening out the skin tone and reducing dark spots.

Ingredients:

1 tablespoon castor oil

1 teaspoon vitamin C powder

1 tablespoon rose water

Instructions:

- Dissolve the vitamin C powder in the rose water, stirring until fully dissolved.

- Add the castor oil to the solution and mix well.

- After cleansing and toning your face, apply 3-4 drops of the serum to your face and neck.

- Gently massage the serum into your skin, focusing on areas with dark spots or sun damage.

- Allow the serum to fully absorb, then apply a moisturizer or sunscreen if using during the day. Vitamin C can make your skin more sensitive to sunlight, so it's important to follow up with SPF during the day.

- Use this serum daily to help brighten your complexion and reduce hyperpigmentation over time.

12. Castor Oil & Green Tea Infusion Anti-Aging Mask

Green tea is packed with antioxidants that help protect the skin from environmental damage and free radicals. Paired with castor oil's hydrating properties, this mask is perfect for rejuvenating and soothing tired, aging skin.

Ingredients:

1 tablespoon castor oil

2 tablespoons brewed green tea (cooled)

1 teaspoon honey

Instructions:

- Brew a cup of green tea and allow it to cool completely.

- In a small bowl, mix the castor oil, cooled green tea, and honey until the ingredients are well combined.

- After cleansing your face, apply a thin, even layer of the mask using your fingers or a brush.

- Let the mask sit for 15-20 minutes, allowing the antioxidants in the green tea to work alongside the hydrating properties of the castor oil.

- Rinse the mask off with lukewarm water, using a soft washcloth to gently wipe away any residue.

- Pat your skin dry and follow up with a light moisturizer. Use this mask once a week to help protect and rejuvenate your skin, leaving it feeling fresh and youthful.

Moisturizing recipes

Each recipe is designed to hydrate and protect the skin, keeping it soft, smooth, and glowing.

13. Castor Oil & Shea Butter Deep Moisturizing Cream

This ultra-rich cream is perfect for dry and rough skin. The combination of castor oil and shea butter provides long-lasting moisture, while lavender essential oil adds a calming touch for both skin and senses. It's ideal for replenishing the skin's barrier and protecting it from harsh elements.

Ingredients:

2 tablespoons castor oil

2 tablespoons shea butter

5 drops lavender essential oil

Instructions:

- Melt the shea butter in a double boiler over low heat until completely liquefied.

- Remove from heat and stir in the castor oil and lavender essential oil until well combined.

- Allow the mixture to cool to room temperature, then place it in the refrigerator for about 30 minutes to solidify.

- Once the mixture has solidified, use a hand mixer to whip it until it reaches a light and fluffy consistency.

- Store the whipped cream in a glass jar with a lid. Apply a small amount to dry areas such as elbows, knees, or heels, massaging in circular motions until fully absorbed. Use after a bath or shower for best results.

14. Castor Oil & Aloe Vera Light Moisturizer

This light moisturizer combines the hydrating properties of castor oil with the soothing benefits of aloe vera, making it perfect for sensitive or irritated skin. Aloe vera's cooling effect helps reduce redness while castor oil locks in moisture without clogging pores.

Ingredients:

2 tablespoons castor oil

2 tablespoons aloe vera gel

5 drops chamomile essential oil

Instructions:

- In a small bowl, mix the castor oil, aloe vera gel, and chamomile essential oil until fully blended.

- After cleansing your face, apply a small amount of the moisturizer to your face and neck, using your fingertips to gently massage it into the skin in upward, circular motions.

- Focus on areas prone to irritation or redness, allowing the mixture to absorb fully into the skin. This light moisturizer is suitable for daily use, morning or night.

- For an extra cooling effect, store the mixture in the fridge before application.

15. Castor Oil & Cocoa Butter Hydrating Balm

This balm offers deep hydration for very dry skin. Cocoa butter softens and nourishes while castor oil helps lock in moisture. It's an excellent solution for tackling cracked heels, elbows, and other problem areas.

Ingredients:

2 tablespoons castor oil

2 tablespoons cocoa butter

1 tablespoon almond oil

Instructions:

- Melt the cocoa butter in a double boiler until completely liquefied.

- Remove from heat and stir in the castor oil and almond oil until fully mixed.

- Pour the mixture into a small glass jar and allow it to cool at room temperature until solid.

- Once solidified, apply a small amount of the balm to dry areas, such as your hands, feet, or elbows.

- Massage the balm into the skin until fully absorbed. For best results, apply before bedtime and wear socks or gloves to enhance hydration overnight.

16. Castor Oil & Coconut Oil Daily Moisturizer

This everyday moisturizer blends castor oil and coconut oil for soft, smooth skin. Coconut oil adds a lightweight feel and extra hydration, making this a perfect option for both body and face.

Ingredients:

2 tablespoons castor oil

2 tablespoons coconut oil

Instructions:

- Melt the coconut oil in a double boiler over low heat, then remove from heat and stir in the castor oil.

- Pour the mixture into a jar and allow it to cool and solidify at room temperature.

- After cleansing your skin, scoop out a small amount of the solidified moisturizer, and rub it between your palms to melt it into an oil.

- Massage the oil into your skin using circular motions, focusing on dry or rough patches.

- Use this moisturizer daily for soft, hydrated skin. It works especially well after a bath or shower to lock in moisture.

17. Castor Oil & Avocado Oil Nourishing Cream

Avocado oil's vitamins A and E work with castor oil to deeply nourish and repair dry or aging skin, making this a highly effective moisturizer. It's especially beneficial for revitalizing dull skin and protecting against environmental damage.

Ingredients:

2 tablespoons castor oil

2 tablespoons avocado oil

1 tablespoon beeswax

Instructions:

- Melt the beeswax in a double boiler over low heat, then remove from heat and stir in the castor oil and avocado oil until well combined.

- Pour the cream mixture into a clean jar and allow it to cool completely at room temperature.

- Once cooled, apply a small amount of the cream to your face and neck, gently massaging it in using upward strokes.

- Use this cream daily for best results, particularly in the evening to allow for overnight skin repair and hydration.

18. Castor Oil & Jojoba Oil Lightweight Moisturizer

Jojoba oil, closely resembling the skin's natural oils, makes this a great lightweight moisturizer, especially for oily or combination skin types. It hydrates without leaving a greasy residue, balancing moisture levels effectively.

Ingredients:

2 tablespoons castor oil

2 tablespoons jojoba oil

5 drops tea tree essential oil (optional)

Instructions:

- In a small bottle, combine the castor oil, jojoba oil, and tea tree essential oil (if using).

- Shake the mixture well before each use.

- After cleansing your face, apply a few drops to your fingertips and gently massage into your skin, focusing on areas prone to oiliness or dryness.

- Use this lightweight moisturizer every morning to help balance your skin's moisture levels without clogging pores.

19. Castor Oil & Vitamin E Hydration Boost Cream

This cream uses vitamin E's antioxidant properties to repair damaged skin while castor oil hydrates and restores moisture. It's especially useful for healing dry patches or irritated skin caused by harsh environmental factors.

Ingredients:

2 tablespoons castor oil

1 tablespoon vitamin E oil

1 tablespoon shea butter

Instructions:

- Melt the shea butter in a double boiler over low heat until fully liquefied.

- Remove from heat and stir in the castor oil and vitamin E oil.

- Pour the mixture into a small jar and allow it to cool and solidify.

- Once solid, scoop out a small amount and warm it between your fingers before applying to dry or irritated areas.

- Massage the cream into your skin until fully absorbed. Use as needed to keep your skin soft and hydrated, especially during colder months.

20. Castor Oil & Olive Oil Ultra-Moisturizing Lotion

Olive oil and castor oil come together in this rich, ultra-moisturizing lotion, perfect for combating dry winter skin. Olive oil's rich antioxidants help protect the skin while castor oil seals in moisture.

Ingredients:

2 tablespoons castor oil

2 tablespoons olive oil

1 tablespoon beeswax

Instructions:

- Melt the beeswax in a double boiler over low heat, then stir in the castor oil and olive oil until fully blended.

- Pour the mixture into a jar and allow it to cool to room temperature.

- After a bath or shower, apply a generous amount of the lotion to your skin, massaging it in with long strokes to help it absorb.

- Use this lotion daily for deeply nourished and protected skin, focusing on particularly dry areas like elbows and knees.

21. Castor Oil & Argan Oil Hydration Serum

Argan oil, rich in essential fatty acids, adds an extra layer of hydration in this lightweight serum, perfect for soft, glowing skin. It's an ideal solution for those looking for a non-greasy, effective serum.

Ingredients:

1 tablespoon castor oil

1 tablespoon argan oil

Instructions:

- In a small dropper bottle, mix the castor oil and argan oil.

- After cleansing your face, apply 2-3 drops of the serum to your fingertips and warm it by rubbing your hands together.

- Gently press the serum into your face, focusing on areas prone to dryness.

- Massage the serum in using upward, circular motions. This serum can be used morning and night for glowing, hydrated skin.

22. Castor Oil & Rose Water Soothing Moisturizer

Rose water calms sensitive skin while castor oil locks in moisture, making this a gentle, soothing moisturizer. It's perfect for daily use, especially if your skin is prone to redness or irritation.

Ingredients:

2 tablespoons castor oil

2 tablespoons rose water

Instructions:

- In a small bowl, mix the castor oil and rose water until fullymixed. Stir thoroughly until combined.

- After cleansing, apply a small amount of the moisturizer to your face and neck. Massage it in gently with your fingertips using circular motions.

- Allow it to absorb fully into your skin. This lightweight moisturizer can be used morning or night for soothing hydration.

23. Castor Oil & Almond Oil Nourishing Body Lotion

Almond oil's emollient properties, combined with castor oil, create a nourishing body lotion that softens and hydrates the skin. It's ideal for keeping your skin moisturized all day, especially in dry or cold conditions.

Ingredients:

2 tablespoons castor oil

2 tablespoons almond oil

1 tablespoon beeswax

Instructions:

- Melt the beeswax in a double boiler over low heat until fully liquefied.

- Remove from heat and stir in the castor oil and almond oil until combined.

- Pour the mixture into a jar and let it cool at room temperature until solidified.

- After bathing, scoop a small amount of the lotion into your hands and warm it between your palms.

- Massage it into your skin, focusing on dry areas like arms, legs, and hands. Use daily to keep your skin soft and hydrated.

24. Castor Oil & Honey Hydration Mask

Honey, a natural humectant, draws moisture into the skin, while castor oil provides hydration and smoothness in this deeply nourishing mask. This combination leaves your skin soft, supple, and glowing.

Ingredients:

2 tablespoons castor oil

1 tablespoon honey

Instructions:

- In a small bowl, mix the castor oil and honey until you get a smooth and even texture.

- After cleansing your face, apply the mask evenly to your skin, avoiding the eye area.

- Let the mask sit for 15-20 minutes to allow the honey to hydrate and the castor oil to nourish your skin.

- Rinse thoroughly with lukewarm water and pat your skin dry with a clean towel.

- Follow up with a light moisturizer to lock in the hydration. Use this mask once or twice a week for glowing, hydrated skin.

Serums and Treatments for Different Skin Types (Dry, Sensitive, Oily)

These serums and treatments are designed to address the specific needs of dry, sensitive, and oily skin types, while leveraging the nourishing and hydrating properties of castor oil. Each recipe provides targeted care to help balance and protect the skin.

25. Castor Oil & Rosehip Oil Serum for Dry Skin

This hydrating serum is perfect for dry skin. Castor oil locks in moisture, while rosehip oil promotes skin regeneration and hydration, making it ideal for reducing flakiness and dryness.

Ingredients:

2 tablespoons castor oil

2 tablespoons rosehip oil

5 drops lavender essential oil

Instructions:

- Combine castor oil, rosehip oil, and lavender essential oil in a small dropper bottle and shake well.

- After cleansing your face, apply 3-4 drops of the serum to your fingertips.

- Gently press the serum into your skin, focusing on dry areas like cheeks and forehead.

- Massage the serum in upward circular motions, allowing it to absorb fully.

- Use this serum daily, especially in the evening, for best hydration results.

26. Castor Oil & Chamomile Serum for Sensitive Skin

This serum is designed to calm sensitive or irritated skin. Castor oil's anti-inflammatory properties combined with chamomile's soothing effect make this an excellent choice for reducing redness and irritation.

Ingredients:

2 tablespoons castor oil

2 tablespoons chamomile oil

5 drops calendula essential oil

Instructions:

- Mix castor oil and chamomile oil in a small bottle, adding the calendula essential oil.

- Shake well before each use.

- After cleansing, apply a small amount to your face, gently pressing the serum into areas prone to sensitivity or redness.

- Massage gently, avoiding any areas of active irritation. Use daily to calm and soothe your skin.

27. Castor Oil & Grapeseed Oil Balancing Serum for Oily Skin

Grapeseed oil is lightweight and helps balance sebum production, making this serum perfect for oily skin. Combined with castor oil, it provides hydration without clogging pores.

Ingredients:

2 tablespoons castor oil

2 tablespoons grapeseed oil

5 drops tea tree essential oil

Instructions:

- In a small bottle, mix the castor oil, grapeseed oil, and tea tree essential oil.

- Shake the mixture well before use.

- After cleansing your face, apply 2-3 drops of the serum to your fingertips and gently press it into your skin.

- Focus on oily areas like the T-zone, massaging the serum in using upward strokes.

- Use this serum morning and night to help regulate oil production and keep your skin balanced.

28. Castor Oil & Jojoba Oil Moisturizing Serum for Dry Skin

Jojoba oil closely resembles the skin's natural oils, making it a perfect addition to this moisturizing serum. Castor oil deeply hydrates, making this combination ideal for dry and flaky skin.

Ingredients:

2 tablespoons castor oil

2 tablespoons jojoba oil

5 drops sandalwood essential oil

Instructions:

- In a small dropper bottle, combine castor oil, jojoba oil, and sandalwood essential oil.

- After cleansing, apply 3-4 drops of the serum to your face, gently massaging it in upward, circular motions.

- Focus on particularly dry areas like the cheeks or forehead.

- Use daily, preferably in the evening, to keep your skin deeply moisturized and soft.

29. Castor Oil & Aloe Vera Gel Treatment for Sensitive Skin

This soothing treatment combines the hydrating properties of castor oil with the calming effects of aloe vera, making it perfect for reducing inflammation and irritation in sensitive skin.

Ingredients:

2 tablespoons castor oil

2 tablespoons aloe vera gel

5 drops chamomile essential oil

Instructions:

- Mix the castor oil, aloe vera gel, and chamomile essential oil in a small bowl.

- Apply a thin layer of the treatment to your skin after cleansing, focusing on areas of redness or irritation.

- Leave it on for 10-15 minutes, then rinse with lukewarm water.

- Use once or twice a week to help calm and hydrate your skin.

30. Castor Oil & Witch Hazel Serum for Oily Skin

Witch hazel is a natural astringent that helps tighten pores and reduce oil production, making this serum perfect for oily skin types.

Ingredients:

2 tablespoons castor oil

2 tablespoons witch hazel

5 drops tea tree essential oil

Instructions:

- In a small bottle, mix castor oil, witch hazel, and tea tree essential oil.

- Shake well before each use.

- After cleansing, apply 2-3 drops of the serum to your fingertips and massage into oily areas like the T-zone.

- Focus on your nose, chin, and forehead, where oil tends to accumulate.

- Use daily to help balance oil production and tighten pores.

31. Castor Oil & Calendula Oil Soothing Serum for Sensitive Skin

Calendula oil is known for its healing and soothing properties, making this serum perfect for sensitive or irritated skin. Castor oil provides deep hydration and helps reduce inflammation.

Ingredients:

2 tablespoons castor oil

2 tablespoons calendula oil

5 drops lavender essential oil

Instructions:

- Mix castor oil, calendula oil, and lavender essential oil in a small dropper bottle.

- Apply a few drops of the serum to your face after cleansing, focusing on areas of redness or irritation.

- Massage gently into the skin, allowing it to fully absorb.

- Use this serum as needed to calm sensitive skin.

32. Castor Oil & Rose Water Hydrating Toner for Dry Skin

This lightweight hydrating toner is perfect for dry skin. Rose water hydrates and refreshes the skin, while castor oil locks in moisture, leaving your skin soft and dewy.

Ingredients:

2 tablespoons castor oil

2 tablespoons rose water

5 drops geranium essential oil

Instructions:

- Mix castor oil, rose water, and geranium essential oil in a spray bottle.

- Shake well before use.

- After cleansing, spritz the toner onto your face or apply it using a cotton pad.

- Gently press the toner into your skin, allowing it to absorb before applying moisturizer.

- Use morning and night to keep your skin hydrated.

33. Castor Oil & Neem Oil Purifying Serum for Oily Skin

Neem oil is known for its antibacterial properties, making this serum ideal for purifying oily skin prone to breakouts. Castor oil provides balanced hydration without clogging pores.

Ingredients:

2 tablespoons castor oil

2 tablespoons neem oil

5 drops tea tree essential oil

Instructions:

- Combine castor oil, neem oil, and tea tree essential oil in a small dropper bottle.

- Shake well before use.

- After cleansing, apply 3-4 drops of the serum to your fingertips and gently press it into oily or acne-prone areas.

- Use light, circular motions to massage it into the skin, focusing on areas prone to breakouts.

- Use daily for clearer, more balanced skin.

34. Castor Oil & Avocado Oil Restorative Treatment for Dry Skin

This restorative treatment provides intense moisture for very dry or damaged skin. Avocado oil is rich in vitamins, while castor oil helps lock in hydration.

Ingredients:

2 tablespoons castor oil

2 tablespoons avocado oil

5 drops frankincense essential oil

Instructions:

- In a small bowl, mix castor oil, avocado oil, and frankincense essential oil.

- After cleansing, apply a small amount of the treatment to dry areas like the cheeks or forehead.

- Massage gently into the skin using circular motions until fully absorbed.

- Use this treatment at night to allow your skin to repair and hydrate overnight.

35. Castor Oil & Lavender Oil Calming Serum for Sensitive Skin

Lavender oil's soothing and calming properties make this serum perfect for sensitive or irritated skin. Combined with castor oil, it provides hydration while reducing redness and inflammation.

Ingredients:

2 tablespoons castor oil

2 tablespoons lavender oil

Instructions:

- Combine the castor oil and lavender oil in a small dropper bottle and shake well.

- After cleansing, apply 2-3 drops of the serum to your face, gently massaging it into your skin with upward motions.

- Focus on areas prone to redness or sensitivity.

- Use this serum daily to help calm and soothe sensitive skin.

36. Castor Oil & Green Tea Extract Clarifying Serum for Oily Skin

Green tea extract is packed with antioxidants that help reduce inflammation and combat acne, making this serum ideal for oily skin. Combined with castor oil, it provides gentle hydration without clogging pores.

Ingredients:

2 tablespoons castor oil

2 tablespoons green tea extract

5 drops lemon essential oil

Instructions:

- In a small dropper bottle, mix the castor oil, green tea extract, and lemon essential oil.

- After cleansing, apply 3-4 drops of the serum to your fingertips and gently press it into your skin, focusing on oily or acne-prone areas.

- Use circular motions to massage the serum into your skin, particularly in the T-zone.

- Use this serum daily to reduce oil production and clarify your skin.

37. Castor Oil & Evening Primrose Oil Healing Serum for Sensitive Skin

Evening primrose oil is known for its anti-inflammatory properties, making it an excellent addition to this healing serum for sensitive skin. Castor oil hydrates and helps repair irritated areas.

Ingredients:

2 tablespoons castor oil

2 tablespoons evening primrose oil

5 drops chamomile essential oil

Instructions:

- Combine castor oil, evening primrose oil, and chamomile essential oil in a small dropper bottle.

- After cleansing, apply a small amount of the serum to your face, focusing on areas prone to redness or irritation.

- Gently massage the serum into your skin in circular motions, allowing it to fully absorb.

- Use daily for calming and healing sensitive skin.

38. Castor Oil & Carrot Seed Oil Brightening Serum for Dry Skin

Carrot seed oil is rich in antioxidants that help brighten the skin and even out skin tone, making this serum perfect for dry and dull skin. Castor oil ensures deep hydration and nourishment.

Ingredients:

2 tablespoons castor oil

2 tablespoons carrot seed oil

5 drops geranium essential oil

Instructions:

- Mix castor oil, carrot seed oil, and geranium essential oil in a small bottle.

- After cleansing, apply 3-4 drops of the serum to your face and neck.

- Massage the serum into your skin using upward strokes, focusing on areas that need brightening or moisture.

- Use this serum at night for best results, allowing it to absorb and work overnight.

39. Castor Oil & Tea Tree Oil Anti-Acne Treatment for Oily Skin

Tea tree oil is widely known for its antibacterial and acne-fighting properties. When combined with castor oil, this treatment helps reduce breakouts and inflammation while keeping the skin hydrated.

Ingredients:

2 tablespoons castor oil

2 tablespoons tea tree oil

Instructions:

- In a small bottle, mix castor oil and tea tree oil together.

- After cleansing, apply 2-3 drops of the treatment to areas prone to acne, such as the chin, nose, or forehead.

- Gently massage the treatment into your skin, focusing on blemished areas.

- Use this treatment nightly to reduce acne and inflammation.

40. Castor Oil & Lavender Calming Treatment for Sensitive Skin

This calming treatment uses lavender oil to reduce redness and irritation while castor oil provides hydration, making it perfect for sensitive skin prone to flare-ups.

Ingredients:

2 tablespoons castor oil

2 tablespoons lavender essential oil

Instructions:

- Mix castor oil and lavender essential oil in a small dropper bottle.

- After cleansing, apply a small amount to your face and gently massage it in with circular motions, focusing on areas prone to redness or irritation.

- Use nightly to help soothe and calm sensitive skin.

Chapter Four

Haircare (20 Recipes)

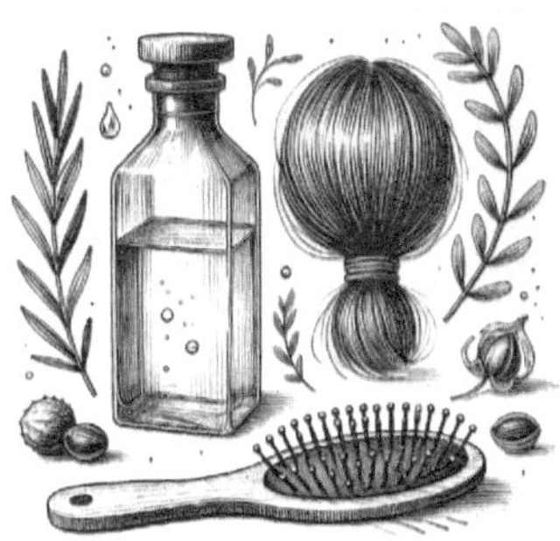

Castor oil is a go-to for hair health, known for promoting growth, thickening thinning hair, and repairing damage. Packed with fatty acids, it nourishes the scalp, boosts circulation, and locks in moisture. In this section, you'll find simple, effective recipes for hair masks, oils, and treatments designed to stimulate growth and restore your hair's strength and shine. Whether you're aiming for longer hair or revitalizing damaged strands, these recipes harness the power of castor oil for optimal results.

41. Castor Oil & Coconut Oil Hair Growth Mask

This mask combines castor oil and coconut oil to nourish the scalp and stimulate hair growth. Coconut oil strengthens hair strands while castor oil boosts circulation to the hair follicles, encouraging thicker, healthier hair. It's a deeply moisturizing treatment that works wonders for brittle or thinning hair.

Ingredients:

2 tablespoons castor oil

2 tablespoons coconut oil

Instructions:

- Melt the coconut oil in a double boiler and mix in the castor oil until well blended.

- Apply the oil mixture to your scalp using your fingertips, massaging gently for 5-10 minutes to promote circulation.

- Work the remaining oil through your hair, focusing on the ends.

- Leave the mask on for at least 30 minutes, or overnight for deeper hydration.

- Rinse thoroughly and shampoo as usual. Use once a week for best results.

42. Castor Oil & Aloe Vera Hair Repair Mask

This repairing hair mask is ideal for damaged or dry hair. Castor oil provides deep hydration, while aloe vera soothes the scalp and helps restore hair softness and shine. This mask also helps improve hair elasticity, making it less prone to breakage.

Ingredients:

2 tablespoons castor oil

2 tablespoons aloe vera gel

1 tablespoon honey

Instructions:

- Mix castor oil, aloe vera gel, and honey in a bowl until well combined.

- Apply the mixture to damp hair, focusing on damaged ends.

- Massage gently into your scalp and work the mask through the length of your hair.

- Let the mask sit for 30 minutes, then rinse thoroughly with lukewarm water and shampoo.

- Use this treatment weekly to repair damaged hair and restore shine.

43. Castor Oil & Rosemary Hair Growth Treatment

Rosemary essential oil is known for stimulating hair growth and improving scalp health. Combined with castor oil, this treatment helps boost hair density and reduces thinning. The potent combination also helps prevent dandruff and scalp irritation.

Ingredients:

2 tablespoons castor oil

10 drops rosemary essential oil

Instructions:

- In a small bowl, mix castor oil and rosemary essential oil until fully blended.

- Using your fingertips, apply the mixture to your scalp, massaging gently in circular motions for 5-10 minutes to stimulate hair follicles.

- Work the oil through the rest of your hair, focusing on the roots.

- Leave the treatment on for at least 30 minutes, or overnight for maximum effect.

- Rinse and shampoo thoroughly. Use this treatment 1-2 times per week for visible hair growth results.

44. Castor Oil & Argan Oil Shine-Boosting Hair Mask

Argan oil is packed with essential fatty acids and vitamin E, which help add shine and smoothness to dull hair. Paired with castor oil, this mask delivers nourishment and luster to your hair. It's ideal for those looking to tame frizz and restore natural hair texture.

Ingredients:

2 tablespoons castor oil

2 tablespoons argan oil

Instructions:

- In a small bowl, combine castor oil and argan oil until fully mixed.

- Apply the oil mixture to your scalp, massaging it in gently to boost circulation.

- Work the remaining oil through the length of your hair, focusing on the ends.

- Leave the mask on for 30 minutes or overnight for an intensive treatment.

- Rinse with warm water and shampoo as usual. Use this mask once a week to maintain shine and softness.

45. Castor Oil & Honey Hair Treatment for Split Ends

This treatment is designed to nourish and repair split ends. Castor oil provides hydration while honey helps seal the hair cuticles, preventing further damage. It's a fantastic option for those with dry or heat-damaged hair.

Ingredients:

2 tablespoons castor oil

1 tablespoon honey

1 egg yolk

Instructions:

- Whisk together castor oil, honey, and egg yolk until smooth.

- Apply the mixture to the ends of your hair, working up to mid-length.

- Gently massage the mixture into your hair, avoiding the scalp.

- Leave the treatment on for 20-30 minutes, then rinse with cool water and shampoo as usual.

- Use once a week to reduce split ends and keep your hair healthy.

46. Castor Oil & Peppermint Oil Scalp Treatment for Hair Growth

Peppermint oil stimulates blood flow to the scalp, encouraging hair growth. When combined with castor oil, this scalp treatment promotes healthier, stronger hair. It also has a cooling effect that soothes itching and dryness.

Ingredients:

2 tablespoons castor oil

10 drops peppermint essential oil

Instructions:

- Mix castor oil and peppermint essential oil in a small bowl.

- Using your fingertips, apply the mixture directly to your scalp, massaging gently in circular motions.

- Work the remaining oil down the length of your hair.

- Leave the treatment on for 30 minutes or overnight for deeper penetration.

- Rinse and shampoo as usual. Use this treatment 1-2 times per week to stimulate hair growth.

47. Castor Oil & Avocado Oil Mask for Dry Hair

This rich, nourishing mask is perfect for dry and damaged hair. Avocado oil adds essential fatty acids and vitamins, while castor oil locks in moisture and hydrates the hair shaft. This treatment revitalizes your hair, leaving it softer and shinier after each use.

Ingredients:

2 tablespoons castor oil

2 tablespoons avocado oil

1 tablespoon coconut oil

Instructions:

- Melt the coconut oil in a double boiler and mix it with castor oil and avocado oil.

- Apply the mixture to damp hair, massaging it into your scalp and working it through to the ends.

- Leave the mask on for 30-40 minutes, then rinse thoroughly with warm water and shampoo.

- Use weekly for deeply hydrated, softer hair.

48. Castor Oil & Olive Oil Treatment for Thinning Hair

Olive oil helps nourish the scalp and hair follicles, while castor oil strengthens hair, reducing thinning and breakage. This treatment is ideal for those experiencing hair loss and thinning, providing essential nutrients to improve hair volume and texture.

Ingredients:

2 tablespoons castor oil

2 tablespoons olive oil

Instructions:

- Mix castor oil and olive oil in a small bowl.

- Using your fingertips, apply the mixture to your scalp, massaging in circular motions for 5-10 minutes.

- Work the oil through the length of your hair, focusing on thinning areas.

- Leave the treatment on for 30 minutes or overnight for deeper results.

- Rinse and shampoo thoroughly. Use this treatment twice a week to promote hair growth.

49. Castor Oil & Egg Hair Mask for Damaged Hair

Eggs are rich in proteins that help repair damaged hair, while castor oil provides moisture and nourishment. This mask strengthens weak strands and promotes healthy hair growth. It also helps to rebuild the hair structure from within, making it more resilient.

Ingredients:

2 tablespoons castor oil

1 egg yolk

1 tablespoon honey

Instructions:

- Whisk together castor oil, egg yolk, and honey until smooth.

- Apply the mixture to your hair, focusing on damaged areas.

- Gently massage the mask into your scalp and work it through your hair.

- Leave it on for 20-30 minutes, then rinse with cool water and shampoo.

- Use this mask once a week to repair and strengthen damaged hair.

50. Castor Oil & Lavender Oil Scalp Soothing Treatment

Lavender essential oil has calming and soothing properties, making this treatment ideal for an irritated or itchy scalp. Combined with castor oil, it provides moisture while calming scalp issues. This treatment also promotes relaxation, making it a perfect part of your self-care routine.

Ingredients:

2 tablespoons castor oil

10 drops lavender essential oil

Instructions:

- In a small bowl, mix castor oil with lavender essential oil.

- Apply the mixture to your scalp, gently massaging it in with your fingertips to soothe irritation.

- Leave the treatment on for 30 minutes or overnight.

- Rinse and shampoo thoroughly. Use once a week for best results in calming scalp irritation.

51. Castor Oil & Almond Oil Hair Strengthening Mask

Almond oil is rich in vitamins and minerals that nourish the hair, while castor oil strengthens and thickens weak strands. Thus, this mask is perfect for those experiencing hair breakage or thinning. Regular use helps maintain healthier, shinier, and stronger hair.

Ingredients:

2 tablespoons castor oil

2 tablespoons almond oil

1 tablespoon honey

Instructions:

- In a bowl, mix castor oil, almond oil, and honey until smooth.

- Apply the mixture to your scalp and hair, focusing on areas that need extra strengthening.

- Massage gently into the scalp for 5 minutes, then work through to the ends of your hair.

- Leave the mask on for 30 minutes or overnight, then rinse thoroughly and shampoo.

- Use this mask once a week to strengthen hair and reduce breakage.

52. Castor Oil & Apple Cider Vinegar Scalp Treatment

Apple cider vinegar is great for clarifying the scalp and balancing its pH, while castor oil provides moisture and nourishment. This treatment is excellent for those with oily scalps or dandruff, as it helps remove product buildup and restore scalp health.

Ingredients:

2 tablespoons castor oil

2 tablespoons apple cider vinegar

1 tablespoon water

Instructions:

- Mix castor oil, apple cider vinegar, and water in a small bowl.

- Using your fingertips, apply the mixture to your scalp, gently massaging it in to stimulate circulation and remove buildup.

- Leave the treatment on for 15-20 minutes, then rinse thoroughly with cool water and shampoo.

- Use once a week to cleanse the scalp and maintain healthy hair.

53. Castor Oil & Hibiscus Hair Growth Mask

Hibiscus is known for its ability to promote hair growth and add shine. Combined with castor oil, this mask nourishes the scalp and encourages healthy hair development. It's particularly beneficial for people with thinning hair or hair prone to breakage.

Ingredients:

2 tablespoons castor oil

1 tablespoon hibiscus powder

1 tablespoon coconut oil

Instructions:

- Melt the coconut oil and mix it with castor oil and hibiscus powder to form a paste.

- Apply the paste to your scalp, massaging it in gently to stimulate hair follicles.

- Work the remaining paste through the length of your hair.

- Leave the mask on for 30-40 minutes, then rinse and shampoo as usual.

- Use this mask weekly to promote hair growth and add shine.

54. Castor Oil & Tea Tree Oil Anti-Dandruff Treatment

Tea tree oil is a powerful natural antifungal that helps fight dandruff, while castor oil hydrates and soothes the scalp. This treatment is perfect for combating flaky or itchy scalps and can help maintain a healthier scalp long-term.

Ingredients:

2 tablespoons castor oil

10 drops tea tree essential oil

Instructions:

- Mix castor oil and tea tree oil in a small bowl.

- Apply the mixture directly to your scalp, massaging gently in circular motions.

- Leave the treatment on for 30 minutes before rinsing and shampooing.

- Use this treatment once a week to eliminate dandruff and keep your scalp healthy.

55. Castor Oil & Avocado Hair Mask for Damaged Hair

This rich hair mask provides deep hydration to damaged hair. Avocado is full of vitamins and fatty acids that repair the hair shaft, while castor oil locks in moisture and nourishes the scalp. This is an ideal treatment for heat-damaged or chemically treated hair.

Ingredients:

2 tablespoons castor oil

1 ripe avocado

1 tablespoon honey

Instructions:

- Mash the avocado in a bowl and mix in the castor oil and honey.

- Apply the mask to damp hair, focusing on the scalp and damaged ends.

- Massage the mixture into your scalp and work through to the tips of your hair.

- Leave the mask on for 30 minutes, then rinse with cool water and shampoo.

- Use this mask weekly to repair and nourish damaged hair.

56. Castor Oil & Banana Hair Moisturizing Mask

Bananas are rich in potassium and vitamins that hydrate and nourish the hair, making this mask ideal for dry and frizzy hair. Castor oil locks in moisture and smooths the hair cuticle, helping reduce frizz and breakage over time.

Ingredients:

2 tablespoons castor oil

1 ripe banana

1 tablespoon olive oil

Instructions:

- Mash the banana in a bowl and mix in the castor oil and olive oil until smooth.

- Apply the mask to damp hair, working it through from the scalp to the ends.

- Let the mask sit for 20-30 minutes, then rinse thoroughly with warm water and shampoo.

- Use this mask once a week to keep your hair hydrated and frizz-free.

57. Castor Oil & Ginger Scalp Stimulation Treatment

Ginger is known for stimulating blood circulation, which helps promote hair growth. Combined with castor oil, this scalp treatment encourages healthier, thicker hair. It's great for reviving slow-growing hair and reducing hair loss due to poor scalp health.

Ingredients:

2 tablespoons castor oil

1 tablespoon grated fresh ginger

Instructions:

- In a small bowl, mix castor oil and freshly grated ginger.

- Apply the mixture to your scalp, gently massaging it in circular motions for 5-10 minutes.

- Leave the treatment on for 20-30 minutes, then rinse thoroughly with water and shampoo.

- Use once a week to stimulate hair growth and improve scalp health.

58. Castor Oil & Onion Juice Hair Growth Treatment

Onion juice is rich in sulfur, which helps boost hair growth and reduce hair thinning. Combined with castor oil, this treatment promotes strong, healthy hair. It also helps improve hair texture and prevent breakage, making it an excellent remedy for thinning hair.

Ingredients:

2 tablespoons castor oil

2 tablespoons onion juice

Instructions:

- Mix castor oil and onion juice in a small bowl.

- Using a cotton ball or your fingertips, apply the mixture to your scalp, focusing on areas with thinning hair.

- Gently massage the mixture into your scalp for 5 minutes.

- Leave the treatment on for 30 minutes before rinsing and shampooing.

- Use this treatment once a week for best results in promoting hair growth.

59. Castor Oil & Vitamin E Hair Treatment

Vitamin E is a powerful antioxidant that repairs damaged hair and protects it from environmental stress. This treatment helps restore moisture and strength to brittle or dry hair. It's particularly effective for those with split ends or dull hair.

Ingredients:

2 tablespoons castor oil

2 vitamin E capsules (pierced for the oil)

Instructions:

- In a small bowl, mix the castor oil with the oil from the vitamin E capsules.

- Apply the mixture to your scalp, massaging it gently to stimulate circulation.

- Work the oil through the length of your hair, focusing on damaged areas.

- Leave the treatment on for 30 minutes, then rinse and shampoo.

- Use this treatment twice a month to strengthen and protect your hair.

60. Castor Oil & Ylang Ylang Hair Growth Oil

Ylang ylang essential oil is known for promoting hair growth and improving scalp health. Combined with castor oil, this treatment helps reduce hair thinning and strengthens hair follicles. The floral scent also provides a refreshing, uplifting experience during application.

Ingredients:

2 tablespoons castor oil

10 drops ylang ylang essential oil

Instructions:

- Mix castor oil and ylang ylang essential oil in a small dropper bottle.

- Apply a few drops of the oil mixture to your scalp, massaging gently to stimulate the hair follicles.

- Leave the oil on for at least 30 minutes or overnight for best results.

- Rinse and shampoo thoroughly. Use this oil 1-2 times per week to encourage hair growth and strengthen hair.

Chapter Five

Health & Wellness (30 Recipes)

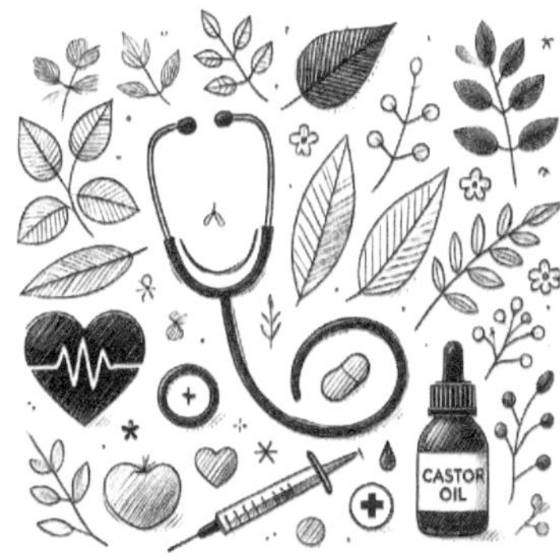

Joint Pain Relief

Joint pain is a common issue, affecting people of all ages due to injury, arthritis, or overuse. Castor oil, known for its anti-inflammatory and pain-relieving properties, has been a natural remedy for joint pain for centuries. The ricinoleic acid in castor oil is particularly effective at reducing inflammation and soothing aching joints. By combining castor oil with other natural ingredients like ginger, cayenne pepper, and essential oils, these recipes are designed to help ease joint discomfort, improve mobility, and promote long-term joint health. Whether you're dealing with arthritis or occasional stiffness, these treatments can provide relief and support healthy joints.

61. Castor Oil & Ginger Warm Compress for Joint Pain

This warm compress combines the anti-inflammatory properties of castor oil with the warming effects of ginger. The heat helps penetrate deep into the joints, providing soothing relief from stiffness and pain. Ginger's natural warmth also promotes blood circulation, which can help alleviate inflammation and support long-term joint health.

Ingredients:

2 tablespoons castor oil

1 tablespoon grated fresh ginger

A soft cloth or gauze

Instructions:

- Warm the castor oil in a small pan over low heat, then stir in the grated ginger.

- Soak the cloth in the mixture and wring it out until damp but not dripping.

- Apply the warm compress to the affected joint, covering it with plastic wrap or a towel to keep the heat in.

- Leave the compress on for 15-20 minutes, then remove and gently massage the area.

- Use this treatment 2-3 times a week to help reduce inflammation and ease joint pain.

62. Castor Oil & Turmeric Anti-Inflammatory Massage Oil

Turmeric contains curcumin, a compound known for its strong anti-inflammatory properties. Combined with castor oil, this massage oil provides relief from joint pain and helps reduce swelling. Turmeric's ability to combat inflammation makes it particularly effective for those with chronic joint pain or arthritis.

Ingredients:

2 tablespoons castor oil

1 teaspoon turmeric powder

5 drops peppermint essential oil

Instructions:

- Mix castor oil and turmeric powder in a small bowl until well combined.

- Heat the mixture slightly to activate the turmeric's properties, then stir in peppermint essential oil for added cooling relief.

- Massage the oil into the affected joint for 5-10 minutes using gentle circular motions.

- Wipe away any excess oil with a warm cloth and allow the area to rest.

- Use daily for ongoing joint pain relief.

63. Castor Oil & Epsom Salt Soak for Joint Pain

Epsom salt is rich in magnesium, which helps relax muscles and reduce inflammation. This soak, combined with castor oil, is ideal for relieving joint stiffness and swelling. The warm water enhances the absorption of magnesium and castor oil, providing deeper pain relief and relaxation.

Ingredients:

2 tablespoons castor oil

1 cup Epsom salt

Warm water (for soaking)

Instructions:

- Fill a large bowl or basin with warm water and add Epsom salt, stirring until dissolved.

- Add the castor oil to the water and mix well.

- Soak the affected joint (hands, feet, elbows) in the solution for 15-20 minutes.

- Pat dry and gently massage the area with a small amount of castor oil.

- Repeat this process 2-3 times a week to reduce pain and swelling.

64. Castor Oil & Cayenne Pepper Pain-Relieving Balm

Cayenne pepper contains capsaicin, which helps block pain signals from reaching the brain. When mixed with castor oil, this balm offers effective relief for joint and muscle pain. The natural heat generated by capsaicin also improves blood flow, which can aid in reducing inflammation over time.

Ingredients:

2 tablespoons castor oil

1 teaspoon cayenne pepper

1 tablespoon beeswax

Instructions:

- Melt the beeswax in a double boiler, then stir in the castor oil and cayenne pepper.

- Once combined, let the mixture cool slightly before transferring it to a small container.

- Apply a small amount of the balm to the painful joint, massaging it in with gentle pressure.

- Use caution with cayenne pepper; avoid contact with eyes and wash hands after application.

- Apply as needed for joint pain relief.

65. Castor Oil & Lavender Calming Compress for Joint Pain

Lavender essential oil is known for its calming and soothing properties. This compress combines lavender with castor oil to relieve both physical joint pain and emotional stress. Lavender's ability to reduce anxiety and stress makes this treatment particularly effective for tension-related joint pain.

Ingredients:

2 tablespoons castor oil

5 drops lavender essential oil

Warm water and a soft cloth

Instructions:

- Mix castor oil and lavender essential oil in a small bowl.

- Soak a soft cloth in warm water, then wring it out.

- Apply the oil mixture to the cloth and place it over the affected joint.

- Leave the compress on for 15-20 minutes, allowing the lavender to calm your senses and the castor oil to reduce inflammation.

- Use this compress 2-3 times a week for both pain and stress relief.

66. Castor Oil & Frankincense Massage Oil for Joint Flexibility

Frankincense is known for its anti-inflammatory and pain-relieving properties, making it a great addition to this massage oil. It helps improve joint flexibility and reduce stiffness, especially for those with arthritis. Regular use can help improve mobility in stiff joints and support overall joint function.

Ingredients:

2 tablespoons castor oil

10 drops frankincense essential oil

Instructions:

- Mix the castor oil and frankincense essential oil in a small bottle.

- Warm the oil slightly before applying it to the affected joint.

- Massage the area with gentle circular motions for 5-10 minutes, focusing on areas of stiffness.

- Use this oil daily to improve joint flexibility and reduce pain.

67. Castor Oil & Clove Oil Warming Joint Relief Treatment

Clove oil contains eugenol, which has anti-inflammatory and pain-relieving properties. This warming treatment, combined with castor oil, helps soothe aching joints and muscles. The heat generated by clove oil also provides instant relief, making it a great option for acute joint pain.

Ingredients:

2 tablespoons castor oil

5 drops clove essential oil

A soft cloth or towel

Instructions:

- Mix castor oil and clove oil in a small bowl and warm it slightly.

- Soak a soft cloth in the oil mixture and wring it out.

- Apply the warm cloth to the painful joint, covering it with a towel to retain heat.

- Leave the treatment on for 20 minutes, then gently massage the area.

- Use this treatment 1-2 times per week for soothing pain relief.

68. Castor Oil & Arnica Gel for Joint Pain and Bruising

Arnica is well-known for its ability to reduce bruising and inflammation. When combined with castor oil, it makes a powerful topical treatment for joints that are painful due to injury or overuse. Arnica's anti-inflammatory properties also help reduce swelling and promote faster healing of injured tissues.

Ingredients:

2 tablespoons castor oil

1 tablespoon arnica gel

Instructions:

- In a small bowl, combine castor oil and arnica gel until well mixed.

- Apply a generous amount to the affected joint, massaging it in gently.

- Allow the mixture to absorb into the skin before covering the area.

- Use this treatment 2-3 times a week to reduce pain and promote healing.

69. Castor Oil & Black Pepper Massage Oil for Joint Stiffness

Black pepper essential oil stimulates circulation and provides a warming sensation that helps relieve joint stiffness. When combined with castor oil, this massage oil helps increase mobility and ease pain. The increased circulation provided by black pepper can also help prevent further stiffness from developing.

Ingredients:

2 tablespoons castor oil

5 drops black pepper essential oil

Instructions:

- Mix castor oil and black pepper essential oil in a small bowl.

- Warm the oil slightly before applying it to the stiff joint.

- Massage the oil into the joint for 5-10 minutes, focusing on increasing blood flow and mobility.

- Repeat as needed to relieve stiffness and improve joint function.

70. Castor Oil & Juniper Oil Detoxifying Massage for Joint Pain

Juniper essential oil helps detoxify the body and reduce inflammation, making it ideal for joint pain relief. Combined with castor oil, this massage oil helps improve circulation and reduce swelling. Its detoxifying properties also support overall joint health, making it beneficial for chronic joint conditions.

Ingredients:

2 tablespoons castor oil

10 drops juniper essential oil

Instructions:

- Mix castor oil and juniper essential oil in a small bowl.

- Massage the oil into the affected joint using firm, circular motions for 5-10 minutes.

- Focus on areas with swelling or inflammation, allowing the oil to absorb fully.

- Use this treatment 2-3 times a week to detoxify and relieve joint pain.

Detox Methods

Detoxifying the body has become a popular practice in holistic wellness as a way to support overall health, improve digestion, and boost energy. Castor oil has been used in detox methods for its ability to stimulate the lymphatic system, encourage circulation, and promote the removal of toxins from the body. These detox recipes incorporate castor oil with other cleansing ingredients like lemon, apple cider vinegar, and essential oils to help flush out impurities and rejuvenate your body. Whether you're looking to cleanse your liver, improve digestion, or simply feel more energized, these castor oil detox methods provide a natural and effective way to support your body's detoxification process.

71. Castor Oil & Lemon Detox Elixir

Lemon is known for its detoxifying properties, particularly for supporting liver function and digestion. When combined with castor oil, this elixir helps to stimulate the lymphatic system and cleanse the body of toxins.

This detox method is ideal for those looking to jumpstart their digestive system and boost their body's natural detox process.

Ingredients:

1 tablespoon castor oil

Juice of 1 fresh lemon

1 cup warm water

Instructions:

- In a glass, mix the castor oil and lemon juice with warm water until well combined.

- Drink this mixture on an empty stomach in the morning to kick-start your detox.

- Follow with plenty of water throughout the day to help flush toxins from the body.

- Repeat this detox method once a week for best results.

72. Castor Oil & Apple Cider Vinegar Cleansing Tonic

Apple cider vinegar is a natural detoxifier known to aid in digestion, improve metabolism, and help flush out toxins. When paired with castor oil, this tonic supports liver function and enhances the body's ability to detoxify itself. This cleansing tonic is perfect for individuals looking for a simple and effective detox solution.

Ingredients:

1 tablespoon castor oil

1 tablespoon apple cider vinegar

1 cup warm water

Instructions:

- Mix castor oil and apple cider vinegar in a glass of warm water, stirring until thoroughly combined.

- **Drink this tonic on an empty stomach** in the morning to maximize its cleansing effects.

- Continue to drink plenty of water throughout the day to help flush toxins from the body.

- Use this tonic 1-2 times a week for best detox results.

73. Castor Oil & Ginger Liver Detox Drink

Ginger has potent anti-inflammatory and detoxifying properties, making it an excellent addition to this liver detox drink. Combined with castor oil, it helps cleanse the liver and improve overall digestion. This drink is great for anyone looking to give their liver a break from processed foods or alcohol.

Ingredients:

1 tablespoon castor oil

1 teaspoon freshly grated ginger

1 cup warm water

Instructions:

- In a small bowl, mix castor oil and freshly grated ginger.

- Pour warm water over the mixture and stir well to combine.

- **Drink this detox mixture on an empty stomach** in the morning to cleanse the liver and stimulate digestion.

- Repeat this detox method once a week for optimal liver health.

74. Castor Oil & Cucumber Detox Water

Cucumber is a natural diuretic and detoxifier that helps flush out toxins and excess water from the body. Paired with castor oil, this detox water helps stimulate the lymphatic system and support overall detoxification. It's a refreshing way to detox and stay hydrated throughout the day.

Ingredients:

1 tablespoon castor oil

1 cucumber (sliced)

1 liter water

Instructions:

- In a large jug, mix castor oil with sliced cucumber and water.

- Stir well and let the mixture sit for at least 30 minutes to allow the cucumber to infuse.

- This detox water can be consumed throughout the day, so no fasting or empty stomach is required.

- Use this method daily during detox programs for best results.

75. Castor Oil & Green Tea Detoxifying Drink

Green tea is packed with antioxidants and is well-known for its detoxifying properties. Combined with castor oil, this drink boosts the body's natural detoxification process and helps to flush out harmful toxins. It's perfect for daily detoxing and supporting a healthy metabolism.

Ingredients:

1 tablespoon castor oil

1 cup brewed green tea

1 teaspoon honey (optional)

Instructions:

- Brew a cup of green tea and let it cool slightly.

- Stir in the castor oil and honey (if using) until well mixed.

- Drink this detoxifying tea on an empty stomach, preferably in the morning, for best detox results.

- Incorporate this drink into your daily routine for ongoing detox-ification support.

76. Castor Oil & Lemon Detox Bath Soak

A detox bath is a great way to relax and cleanse the body from the outside in. Lemon has natural detoxifying properties, and when combined with castor oil, this bath soak helps draw out toxins from the skin and improve circulation. It's ideal for anyone looking to refresh both body and mind.

Ingredients:

2 tablespoons castor oil

Juice of 1 fresh lemon

1 cup Epsom salt

Warm bathwater

Instructions:

- Fill your bathtub with warm water and add castor oil, lemon juice, and Epsom salt.

- Stir the water to ensure the ingredients are well mixed.

- Simply soak in the detox bath for 20-30 minutes, allowing your body to relax and absorb the detoxifying benefits.

- Use this bath once a week to support your body's detoxification process.

77. Castor Oil & Apple Detox Drink

Apples are rich in fiber and pectin, which help bind toxins in the digestive system and promote their elimination. When combined with castor oil, this drink enhances the body's ability to cleanse and detoxify the digestive tract. It's an easy and tasty way to support daily detox.

Ingredients:

1 tablespoon castor oil

1 apple (juiced)

1 teaspoon cinnamon (optional)

Instructions:

- Juice the apple and mix it with castor oil and cinnamon (if using).

- Drink this detox drink on an empty stomach in the morning to cleanse the digestive system.

- Follow up with plenty of water throughout the day to help the body flush out toxins.

- Use this detox method daily for a gentle cleanse.

78. Castor Oil & Aloe Vera Detox Drink

Aloe vera is well-known for its digestive and detoxifying benefits. Paired with castor oil, this drink supports digestion and helps cleanse the colon. This detox drink is particularly beneficial for those experiencing digestive issues or sluggish digestion.

Ingredients:

1 tablespoon castor oil

1 tablespoon aloe vera gel

1 cup warm water

Instructions:

- In a glass, mix castor oil and aloe vera gel with warm water.

- Drink the mixture on an empty stomach in the morning for best detoxifying results.

- Continue to drink water throughout the day to help flush out toxins.

- Use this drink 1-2 times a week to support healthy digestion and detoxification.

79. Castor Oil & Parsley Detox Smoothie

Parsley is a natural diuretic that helps flush out toxins and reduce water retention. Combined with castor oil, this detox smoothie boosts digestion and helps cleanse the body of harmful substances. It's perfect for a morning detox or as part of a healthy detox diet.

Ingredients:

1 tablespoon castor oil

1 cup fresh parsley

1 cucumber (chopped)

1 cup water

Instructions:

- Blend the parsley, cucumber, and water until smooth.

- Stir in the castor oil and mix well.

- This smoothie does not require an empty stomach and can be consumed throughout the day.

- Use this detox smoothie 2-3 times a week for best results.

80. Castor Oil & Flaxseed Detox Cleanse

Flaxseeds are rich in fiber and omega-3 fatty acids, making them excellent for supporting digestion and detoxifying the body. When combined with castor oil, this detox cleanse helps flush out toxins and improve gut health. It's a great way to kickstart your detox journey.

Ingredients:

1 tablespoon castor oil

1 tablespoon ground flaxseeds

1 cup water

Instructions:

- In a glass, mix castor oil and ground flaxseeds with water.

- Drink this cleanse on an empty stomach in the morning for best results in flushing toxins from the digestive system.

- Follow with plenty of water throughout the day to help flush out toxins.

- Use this detox cleanse once a week for best results.

Castor Oil Packs

Castor oil packs are one of the most well-known applications of castor oil for health and wellness. These packs are applied externally and have been traditionally used to relieve pain, reduce inflammation, and support healing. Castor oil packs work by penetrating deep into the skin to improve circulation, stimulate the lymphatic system, and promote tissue repair. Often combined with heat, these packs are commonly used for conditions like joint pain, digestive issues, and menstrual cramps. Easy to make at home, castor oil packs are a versatile and powerful tool for naturally enhancing your body's healing abilities.

81. Basic Castor Oil Pack for Digestive Health

Castor oil packs are known for their ability to support digestive health by stimulating the lymphatic system and reducing inflammation. This basic castor oil pack can help relieve constipation, bloating, and digestive discomfort.

Ingredients:

2-3 tablespoons castor oil

A large piece of flannel or cotton cloth

Plastic wrap

Heating pad or hot water bottle

Instructions:

- Soak the cloth in castor oil until it is saturated but not dripping.

- Place the cloth over your abdomen, focusing on the stomach or lower intestine area.

- Cover the cloth with plastic wrap to prevent the oil from leaking.

- Place a heating pad or hot water bottle over the plastic wrap to warm the castor oil and promote absorption.

- Leave the pack on for 45 minutes to 1 hour, then remove and wipe the area clean.

- Use this castor oil pack 2-3 times a week to support digestive health.

82. Castor Oil & Lemon Balm Pack for Liver Detox

Lemon balm is known for its soothing and detoxifying effects, particularly for the liver. By combining castor oil and lemon balm, this pack promotes liver detox and can help boost your energy levels while supporting overall detoxification.

Ingredients:

2-3 tablespoons castor oil

5 drops lemon balm essential oil

A large piece of flannel or cotton cloth

Plastic wrap

Heating pad or hot water bottle

Instructions:

- Mix the castor oil with lemon balm essential oil and saturate the cloth.

- Apply to the liver area (right side of your abdomen, just below the rib cage).

- Cover with plastic wrap and apply heat for 1 hour.

- Repeat 2-3 times a week for best detox results.

83. Castor Oil & Chamomile Relaxation Pack

Chamomile essential oil is known for its calming effects, helping reduce stress and tension. When combined with castor oil in this pack, it works wonders for easing muscle tightness, calming nerves, and promoting overall relaxation.

Ingredients:

2-3 tablespoons castor oil

5 drops chamomile essential oil

A large piece of flannel or cotton cloth

Plastic wrap

Heating pad or hot water bottle

Instructions:

- Combine castor oil and chamomile oil.

- Saturate the cloth in the mixture and place it on your abdomen or lower back.

- Cover with plastic wrap and apply heat for 45 minutes to 1 hour.

- Use this pack as needed to alleviate stress and muscle tension.

84. Castor Oil & Clary Sage Pack for Menstrual Cramps

Clary sage essential oil is known for its ability to balance hormones and reduce menstrual discomfort. When added to a castor oil pack, it helps to relieve menstrual cramps and support hormonal balance during your cycle.

Ingredients:

2-3 tablespoons castor oil

5 drops clary sage essential oil

A large piece of flannel or cotton cloth

Plastic wrap

Heating pad or hot water bottle

Instructions:

- Mix the castor oil and clary sage essential oil.

- Soak the cloth in the mixture and place it over your lower abdomen.

- Cover with plastic wrap and apply a heating pad or hot water bottle for warmth.

- Leave the pack on for 45 minutes to 1 hour, then clean the area.

- Use during your menstrual cycle to alleviate cramps.

85. Castor Oil & Thyme Pack for Respiratory Health

Thyme is a powerful herb that has natural antimicrobial and decongestant properties. When used in a castor oil pack, it can help alleviate respiratory congestion and support the healing of chest colds or bronchitis.

Ingredients:

2-3 tablespoons castor oil

5 drops thyme essential oil

A large piece of flannel or cotton cloth

Plastic wrap

Heating pad or hot water bottle

Instructions:

- Mix castor oil with thyme essential oil.

- Soak the cloth in the mixture and place it on your chest.

- Cover with plastic wrap and apply heat for 45 minutes to 1 hour.

- Use this pack when dealing with colds or respiratory discomfort.

86. Castor Oil & Rosemary Pack for Headache Relief

Rosemary essential oil helps stimulate circulation and relieve headaches, especially those caused by tension. This pack, using both castor oil and rosemary oil, provides a soothing, relaxing treatment for reducing headache symptoms.

Ingredients:

2 tablespoons castor oil

5 drops rosemary essential oil

A small piece of flannel or cotton cloth

Plastic wrap

Heating pad or hot water bottle

Instructions:

- Combine castor oil and rosemary essential oil.

- Soak the cloth in the mixture and place it on your neck or forehead.

- Cover with plastic wrap and apply heat for 30-45 minutes.

- Use this pack as needed to relieve headaches or tension.

87. Castor Oil & Marjoram Pack for Joint Pain Relief

Marjoram essential oil is known for its ability to reduce pain and inflammation in the joints. By combining it with castor oil in this pack, you can experience enhanced relief from joint stiffness and discomfort, especially for conditions like arthritis.

Ingredients:

2-3 tablespoons castor oil

5 drops marjoram essential oil

A large piece of flannel or cotton cloth

Plastic wrap

Heating pad or hot water bottle

Instructions:

- Mix castor oil with marjoram essential oil.

- Soak the cloth in the mixture and apply it to the affected joint.

- Cover with plastic wrap and apply heat for 45 minutes to 1 hour.

- Use this pack 2-3 times a week for joint pain relief.

88. Castor Oil & Arnica Pack for Muscle Strain Recovery

Arnica is a powerful remedy for reducing muscle pain and inflammation, especially after injury or strain. Combining arnica with castor oil in this pack promotes faster muscle recovery and helps reduce pain from overuse or injury.

Ingredients:

2-3 tablespoons castor oil

1 tablespoon arnica gel

A large piece of flannel or cotton cloth

Plastic wrap

Heating pad or hot water bottle

Instructions:

- Mix castor oil and arnica gel.

- Soak the cloth in the mixture and apply it to the strained muscle.

- Cover with plastic wrap and apply a heating pad or hot water bottle for 45 minutes to 1 hour.

- Use as needed to reduce muscle pain and promote faster recovery.

89. Castor Oil & Basil Pack for Inflammation Reduction

Basil essential oil has anti-inflammatory properties and helps relieve pain in inflamed areas. This pack is perfect for reducing inflammation in the back, joints, or muscles, especially for chronic conditions.

Ingredients:

2-3 tablespoons castor oil

5 drops basil essential oil

A large piece of flannel or cotton cloth

Plastic wrap

Heating pad or hot water bottle

Instructions:

- Mix castor oil with basil essential oil.

- Soak the cloth in the mixture and apply to the inflamed area.

- Cover with plastic wrap and apply heat for 45 minutes to 1 hour.

- Repeat 2-3 times a week to reduce inflammation and relieve pain.

90. Castor Oil & Helichrysum Pack for Healing and Regeneration

Helichrysum essential oil is known for its regenerative properties, making it ideal for promoting tissue healing and reducing scarring. This pack, used with castor oil, is great for healing wounds, scars, and damaged skin.

Ingredients:

2-3 tablespoons castor oil

5 drops helichrysum essential oil

A large piece of flannel or cotton cloth

Plastic wrap

Heating pad or hot water bottle

Instructions:

- Mix castor oil and helichrysum essential oil.

- Soak the cloth in the mixture and apply to the affected area.

- Cover with plastic wrap and apply heat for 45 minutes to 1 hour.

- Use this pack 2-3 times a week to promote healing and reduce scarring.

Chapter Six

Beauty (33 Recipes)

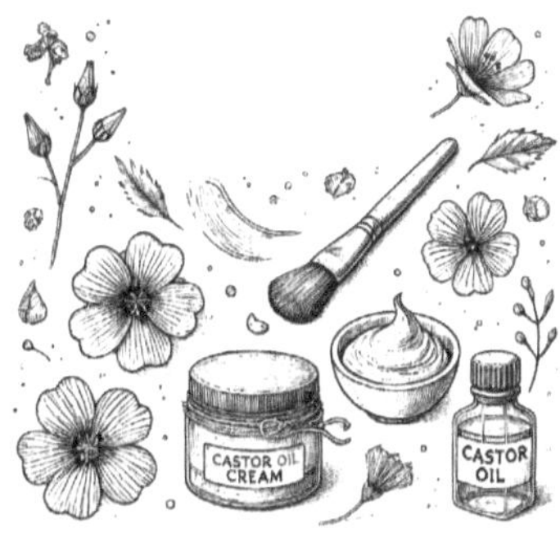

In the world of natural beauty, castor oil has emerged as a star ingredient due to its nourishing, moisturizing, and healing properties. This section explores how castor oil can be used in various DIY beauty products that you can easily make at home, offering a healthier alternative to chemical-laden commercial products. Whether you're looking to craft your own makeup, lip balms, or serums for lash and brow growth, these recipes will help you achieve a radiant look while using natural ingredients.

From creating simple, skin-friendly makeup products to enhancing your lashes and brows with nutrient-rich serums, castor oil is versatile and gentle enough to use daily. It hydrates, promotes hair growth, and protects the skin from environmental stressors, making it a perfect base for beauty recipes that are both effective and free from harmful chemicals.

Now, let's dive into the first set of recipes, beginning with **DIY Makeup**.

DIY Makeup.

91. Castor Oil & Cocoa Powder DIY Foundation

This natural foundation is made from simple ingredients and can be adjusted to match your skin tone by varying the amount of cocoa powder. Castor oil provides hydration while giving the foundation a smooth, creamy texture, ensuring your skin stays moisturized throughout the day. This recipe is perfect for those looking for light coverage that enhances their natural complexion without clogging pores.

Ingredients:

2 tablespoons castor oil

1 tablespoon arrowroot powder

1/2 teaspoon cocoa powder (adjust for skin tone)

1/2 teaspoon cinnamon powder (optional for a warmer tone)

Instructions:

- In a small bowl, mix the arrowroot powder and cocoa powder until well combined.

- Gradually stir in castor oil until you reach a creamy, smooth consistency.

- Adjust the cocoa powder as needed to match your skin tone.

- Apply the foundation with a makeup sponge or brush. Store in an airtight container for up to 3 weeks.

92. Castor Oil & Beetroot Powder DIY Blush

This natural blush gives your cheeks a radiant flush of color while nourishing the skin with castor oil's moisturizing properties. Beetroot powder provides a beautiful natural pigment, giving your cheeks a healthy glow without clogging pores or irritating sensitive skin. This DIY blush is ideal for achieving a fresh, youthful look, perfect for all skin types.

Ingredients:

1 tablespoon castor oil

1 teaspoon beetroot powder (adjust for color intensity)

1 teaspoon arrowroot powder

Instructions:

- In a small bowl, mix the beetroot powder and arrowroot powder together.

- Slowly add castor oil, stirring until the mixture forms a smooth, paste-like consistency.

- Apply a small amount to your cheeks and blend it out with your fingertips or a brush.

- Store in a small container and use within 2-3 weeks.

93. Castor Oil & Activated Charcoal DIY Mascara

This DIY mascara uses the thick, nourishing qualities of castor oil to help lengthen and strengthen lashes, while activated charcoal provides a rich, dark pigment. The combination of ingredients also promotes healthier lash growth, making it a dual-purpose product that enhances your lashes while encouraging thickness and strength. It's an all-natural alternative to conventional mascaras, free of harmful chemicals.

Ingredients:

1 tablespoon castor oil

1 teaspoon activated charcoal

1/2 teaspoon beeswax (for thickening)

Instructions:

- Melt the beeswax in a double boiler, then stir in castor oil and activated charcoal until fully combined.

- Pour the mixture into a clean mascara tube or small container and let it cool.

- Use a clean mascara wand to apply. This mascara nourishes lashes while providing natural, buildable coverage.

- Store for up to 2 months in a cool place.

94. Castor Oil & Arrowroot Powder DIY Translucent Setting Powder

This translucent powder helps to set makeup and reduce shine. Castor oil provides a light moisturizing effect, while arrowroot absorbs excess oil, leaving your skin with a smooth, matte finish. It's an excellent natural alternative to store-bought powders, and it helps keep your makeup in place throughout the day without drying out your skin. Ideal for controlling shine on oily skin, this powder works for all skin types.

Ingredients:

1 tablespoon arrowroot powder

1/4 teaspoon castor oil

A few drops of lavender essential oil (optional)

Instructions:

- In a small bowl, mix the arrowroot powder and castor oil until well combined.

- Add a few drops of lavender essential oil for a calming scent, if desired.

- Apply the powder with a fluffy makeup brush after applying foundation to set your makeup.

- Store in a small container for up to 3 weeks.

95. Castor Oil & Cocoa Butter DIY Contour Stick

This creamy contour stick is perfect for adding definition to your face. The rich texture of cocoa butter, combined with castor oil, makes this contour stick easy to blend for a natural, sculpted look. It provides a smooth, long-lasting finish that nourishes your skin while allowing you to highlight and contour your features with ease. This versatile stick can also double as a bronzer for a sun-kissed glow.

Ingredients:

1 tablespoon castor oil

1 tablespoon cocoa butter (melted)

1 teaspoon cocoa powder (adjust for skin tone)

1/2 teaspoon arrowroot powder

Instructions:

- In a small bowl, mix the cocoa butter and castor oil until smooth.

- Add the cocoa powder and arrowroot powder, stirring until you achieve the desired color and consistency.

- Pour the mixture into an empty lipstick or contour stick container and let it cool and solidify.

- Apply under cheekbones, jawline, and along the nose, blending with a brush or fingertips.

96. Castor Oil & Mica Powder DIY Highlighter

This simple highlighter recipe adds a radiant glow to your skin. Mica powder gives the highlighter a shimmery finish, while castor oil keeps it smooth and hydrating. It's the perfect addition to your makeup routine, offering a luminous, dewy effect without the use of harsh chemicals or artificial ingredients. Ideal for enhancing your cheekbones, brow bone, and other high points of your face.

Ingredients:

1 tablespoon castor oil

1 teaspoon mica powder (choose your preferred shade)

1/2 teaspoon beeswax (optional for thicker texture)

Instructions:

- Melt the beeswax in a double boiler if you prefer a thicker highlighter.

- Stir in the castor oil and mica powder until fully combined.

- Pour the mixture into a small container and let it cool.

- Dab the highlighter on the high points of your face, such as the cheekbones, brow bone, and nose, and blend gently.

97. Castor Oil & Cocoa Butter DIY Lipstick

This DIY lipstick offers rich color with the moisturizing benefits of castor oil and cocoa butter. It provides a creamy texture that hydrates your lips while delivering long-lasting color. By adjusting the beetroot or cocoa powder, you can create custom shades that suit your skin tone while keeping your lips soft and supple all day.

Ingredients:

1 tablespoon castor oil

1 tablespoon cocoa butter

1 teaspoon beetroot powder or cocoa powder (for pigment)

1/2 teaspoon beeswax (optional for a firmer texture)

Instructions:

- Melt cocoa butter and beeswax in a double boiler.

- Stir in castor oil and beetroot or cocoa powder until the mixture is smooth.

- Pour into a lipstick mold or small container and let it cool.

- Apply with a brush or directly from the container for a rich, hydrating color.

98. Castor Oil & Mica Powder DIY Eyeshadow

This eyeshadow recipe combines castor oil with mica powder for a smooth, long-lasting eyeshadow that nourishes your eyelids. Mica powder offers a range of colors and a subtle shimmer. This DIY eyeshadow is ideal for creating a soft, natural look or a more dramatic, bold style depending on the shade of mica powder you choose.

Ingredients:

1 tablespoon castor oil

1 teaspoon mica powder (choose your color)

1/2 teaspoon arrowroot powder (optional for a matte finish)

Instructions:

- In a small bowl, mix mica powder and arrowroot powder.

- Stir in castor oil until the mixture forms a smooth paste.

- Apply to your eyelids using a brush or fingertips for a natural, shimmery look.

- Store in a small container for up to a month.

99. Castor Oil & Cornstarch DIY Face Primer

This lightweight primer helps create a smooth canvas for your makeup by filling in pores and fine lines. Castor oil hydrates the skin, while cornstarch helps control oil and reduce shine throughout the day. This all-natural primer is great for extending the wear of your makeup while giving your skin a soft, dewy glow.

Ingredients:

1 tablespoon castor oil

1 teaspoon cornstarch

1/4 teaspoon aloe vera gel (optional)

Instructions:

- In a small bowl, mix castor oil, cornstarch, and aloe vera gel until smooth.

- Apply a thin layer to your face before applying foundation or concealer.

- Allow it to absorb for a few minutes before continuing with your makeup routine.

100. Castor Oil & Shea Butter DIY Tinted Moisturizer

This tinted moisturizer provides light coverage while deeply hydrating the skin. The combination of shea butter and castor oil creates a creamy formula that evens skin tone and leaves a dewy finish. It's perfect for everyday use, offering both hydration and subtle coverage for a natural, glowing complexion.

Ingredients:

1 tablespoon castor oil

1 tablespoon shea butter

1/2 teaspoon cocoa powder (adjust for skin tone)

Instructions:

- Melt the shea butter in a double boiler and mix it with castor oil.

- Gradually stir in cocoa powder until you reach your desired tint.

- Apply the tinted moisturizer to your face using your fingers or a makeup sponge.

- Store in a small container and use daily for a fresh, natural look.

101. Castor Oil & Aloe Vera DIY BB Cream

This BB cream offers lightweight coverage while also moisturizing, soothing, and protecting your skin. Castor oil and aloe vera work together to create a hydrating, multitasking beauty balm. It's ideal for those who want a minimal makeup look that still evens out the skin tone and provides a radiant glow.

Ingredients:

1 tablespoon castor oil

1 tablespoon aloe vera gel

1 teaspoon arrowroot powder

1/2 teaspoon cocoa powder (optional for tint)

Instructions:

- Mix castor oil, aloe vera gel, and arrowroot powder in a small bowl.

- Stir in cocoa powder for a tinted effect if desired.

- Apply to your face as a light, all-in-one moisturizer and foundation.

- Store in an airtight container and use as part of your daily beauty routine.

102. Castor Oil & Matcha DIY Green Concealer

Matcha powder is perfect for creating a green concealer that neutralizes redness, while castor oil ensures that your skin stays hydrated and soothed throughout the day. This DIY green concealer is excellent for reducing the appearance of blemishes, rosacea, and redness around the nose or cheeks.

Ingredients:

1 tablespoon castor oil

1/2 teaspoon matcha green tea powder

1/2 teaspoon arrowroot powder

Instructions:

- Mix castor oil, matcha powder, and arrowroot powder in a small bowl.

- Apply the green concealer to areas of redness before applying foundation.

- Blend gently with your fingertips or a makeup sponge for smooth coverage.

103. Castor Oil & Beeswax DIY Eyeliner

This DIY eyeliner offers a smooth, rich texture while nourishing your eyelids with castor oil. Beeswax helps thicken the mixture, ensuring it stays in place for hours. The result is a rich, long-lasting eyeliner that is gentle on the delicate skin around the eyes while providing a bold definition.

Ingredients:

1 tablespoon castor oil

1 teaspoon activated charcoal

1/2 teaspoon beeswax

Instructions:

- Melt the beeswax in a double boiler and stir in castor oil and activated charcoal.

- Pour the mixture into a small container and let it cool.

- Apply using an eyeliner brush for precise, long-lasting definition.

104. Castor Oil & Shea Butter DIY Lip and Cheek Tint

This versatile product works as both a lip tint and a cheek blush. The combination of castor oil and shea butter keeps your skin and lips hydrated, while the natural pigment adds a healthy, glowing color. It's perfect for achieving a cohesive, natural look that enhances your skin's natural radiance.

Ingredients:

1 tablespoon castor oil

1 tablespoon shea butter

1 teaspoon beetroot powder or cocoa powder (for color)

Instructions:

- Melt shea butter in a double boiler and mix with castor oil.

- Stir in the beetroot or cocoa powder for the desired color intensity.

- Apply to your lips or dab onto your cheeks for a natural, glowing look.

105. Castor Oil & Cinnamon DIY Bronzer

This bronzer adds a sun-kissed glow to your skin using natural ingredients. Castor oil provides a smooth application, while cinnamon and cocoa powder give you a warm, bronzed finish. Perfect for contouring or adding warmth to your complexion, this DIY bronzer is a healthy, natural alternative to store-bought options.

Ingredients:

1 tablespoon castor oil

1 teaspoon cocoa powder

1/2 teaspoon cinnamon powder

Instructions:

- In a small bowl, mix cocoa powder and cinnamon with castor oil until smooth.

- Apply to the high points of your face, such as your forehead, cheekbones, and nose, using a makeup brush for a sun-kissed effect.

- Blend well for a natural, warm glow.

Lip Balm Recipes

106. Castor Oil & Honey Lip Balm

This rich, moisturizing lip balm combines the hydrating properties of castor oil with the soothing benefits of honey. Together, they create a balm that keeps your lips soft and nourished, ideal for everyday use. Honey also helps lock in moisture and heal chapped lips, making it perfect for dry weather conditions.

Ingredients:

1 tablespoon castor oil

1 teaspoon honey

1/2 teaspoon beeswax

1/2 teaspoon shea butter

Instructions:

- Melt the beeswax and shea butter in a double boiler.

- Stir in castor oil and honey until the mixture is smooth.

- Pour the mixture into a small container and let it cool.

- Apply to your lips throughout the day for long-lasting hydration.

107. Castor Oil & Peppermint Lip Balm

Peppermint essential oil adds a refreshing, cooling sensation to this lip balm while castor oil provides deep hydration. This balm is perfect for soothing dry or cracked lips, especially in the winter months when your lips need extra care. The minty aroma also gives it an invigorating touch.

Ingredients:

1 tablespoon castor oil

1 teaspoon beeswax

5 drops peppermint essential oil

1/2 teaspoon coconut oil

Instructions:

- Melt the beeswax and coconut oil in a double boiler.

- Stir in castor oil and peppermint essential oil until well combined.

- Pour the mixture into a lip balm tube or small container and let it cool.

- Use regularly to keep your lips soft and smooth.

108. Castor Oil & Vanilla Lip Balm

This lip balm offers a sweet, subtle vanilla scent while providing your lips with deep moisture. Castor oil keeps lips hydrated, while vanilla extract adds a comforting aroma. The addition of beeswax ensures the balm stays on your lips for hours, creating a protective barrier.

Ingredients:

1 tablespoon castor oil

1/2 teaspoon vanilla extract

1 teaspoon beeswax

1/2 teaspoon cocoa butter

Instructions:

- Melt the beeswax and cocoa butter in a double boiler.

- Stir in castor oil and vanilla extract until the mixture is smooth.

- Pour into a small tin or container and let it cool completely.

- Apply whenever your lips need a moisturizing boost.

109. Castor Oil & Lemon Lip Balm

Lemon essential oil adds a bright, citrusy scent to this lip balm, while castor oil deeply hydrates the lips. This balm is perfect for brightening your day with its refreshing scent, and the combination of ingredients provides long-lasting moisture and protection for your lips.

Ingredients:

1 tablespoon castor oil

1/2 teaspoon beeswax

5 drops lemon essential oil

1/2 teaspoon shea butter

Instructions:

- Melt the beeswax and shea butter in a double boiler.

- Stir in castor oil and lemon essential oil until well blended.

- Pour the mixture into a lip balm tube or small jar and let it cool.

- Use as needed to keep your lips soft, smooth, and refreshed.

110. Castor Oil & Rose Lip Balm

This luxurious lip balm combines castor oil with the delicate scent of rose essential oil. Rose oil provides soothing properties that calm irritation, while castor oil hydrates and protects your lips from drying out. It's a perfect lip balm for everyday wear or special occasions.

Ingredients:

1 tablespoon castor oil

5 drops rose essential oil

1/2 teaspoon beeswax

1/2 teaspoon coconut oil

Instructions:

- Melt the beeswax and coconut oil in a double boiler.

- Stir in castor oil and rose essential oil until fully combined.

- Pour into a small container and let it cool.

- Apply throughout the day for soft, scented lips.

111. Castor Oil & Cocoa Lip Balm

This nourishing lip balm combines castor oil with the rich, chocolatey scent of cocoa powder. Cocoa butter adds extra moisture and softness, making this balm perfect for dry, cracked lips. The subtle hint of cocoa makes it a deliciously fragrant option for everyday use.

Ingredients:

1 tablespoon castor oil

1/2 teaspoon cocoa butter

1 teaspoon beeswax

1/2 teaspoon cocoa powder

Instructions:

- Melt the beeswax and cocoa butter in a double boiler.

- Stir in castor oil and cocoa powder until smooth.

- Pour the mixture into a small tin and let it cool completely.

- Apply to your lips for a chocolate-scented treat that hydrates and protects.

112. Castor Oil & Lavender Lip Balm

Lavender essential oil provides calming, soothing effects, making this lip balm perfect for relaxation and stress relief. Castor oil offers lasting hydration, while beeswax locks in moisture, ensuring your lips stay soft and protected for hours.

Ingredients:

- 1 tablespoon castor oil

- 5 drops lavender essential oil

- 1 teaspoon beeswax

- 1/2 teaspoon shea butter

Instructions:

- Melt the beeswax and shea butter in a double boiler.

- Stir in castor oil and lavender essential oil until well combined.

- Pour into a lip balm container and let it cool.

- Use daily for soothing hydration with a calming lavender scent.

113. Castor Oil & Grapefruit Lip Balm

This citrusy lip balm combines the refreshing scent of grapefruit essential oil with the moisturizing benefits of castor oil. It's a perfect choice for energizing your senses while keeping your lips soft and supple.

Ingredients:

1 tablespoon castor oil

5 drops grapefruit essential oil

1 teaspoon beeswax

1/2 teaspoon coconut oil

Instructions:

- Melt the beeswax and coconut oil in a double boiler.

- Stir in castor oil and grapefruit essential oil until smooth.

- Pour the mixture into a small container and let it cool.

- Apply for a refreshing, hydrating experience throughout the day.

114. Castor Oil & Almond Lip Balm

This lip balm combines the sweet, nutty aroma of almond oil with the deep hydration of castor oil. The rich blend provides long-lasting moisture and protection, making it a great option for soothing chapped lips, especially during colder months.

Ingredients:

- 1 tablespoon castor oil

- 1 teaspoon almond oil

- 1 teaspoon beeswax

- 1/2 teaspoon shea butter

Instructions:

- Melt the beeswax and shea butter in a double boiler.

- Stir in castor oil and almond oil until the mixture is smooth.

- Pour into a small tin or jar and let it cool.

- Use whenever your lips need extra hydration and protection.

Lash & Brow Growth Serums

115. Castor Oil & Vitamin E Lash Growth Serum

Vitamin E is well known for its ability to nourish and repair hair follicles, making it an excellent addition to this serum for promoting lash growth. Combined with castor oil, it helps thicken and lengthen lashes over time.

Ingredients:

1 tablespoon castor oil

1/2 teaspoon vitamin E oil

Clean mascara wand or small dropper bottle

Instructions:

- In a small bowl, mix the castor oil and vitamin E oil thoroughly until fully combined.

- Transfer the mixture into a clean mascara tube or dropper bottle for easy application.

- Before applying the serum, make sure your lashes are clean and free of makeup. Use a clean mascara wand or dropper to gently coat your lashes from the roots to the tips.

- Be careful not to overload the brush or dropper to avoid oil dripping into your eyes.

- Apply nightly before bed and leave the serum on overnight to allow it to fully absorb into the hair follicles.

- Wash your face as usual in the morning. Use this serum consistently for at least 4-6 weeks to see results.

116. Castor Oil & Aloe Vera Brow Growth Serum

Aloe vera helps to soothe and nourish the skin around the brows while promoting healthier hair growth. Combined with castor oil, this serum encourages fuller, thicker eyebrows.

Ingredients:

1 tablespoon castor oil

1 tablespoon aloe vera gel

Clean brow brush or small dropper bottle

Instructions:

- In a small bowl, mix the castor oil and aloe vera gel until the ingredients are evenly blended.

- Transfer the mixture to a clean dropper bottle or use a clean brow brush for application.

- Before applying, cleanse your eyebrows to remove any oils or makeup.

- Use the dropper or brow brush to apply the serum to the brow area, focusing on sparse spots. Gently massage the serum into the skin around your eyebrows to ensure it penetrates the follicles.

- Allow the serum to sit on your brows overnight, as the castor oil and aloe vera work together to nourish the follicles.

- Wash your face the next morning and continue using daily for fuller brows.

117. Castor Oil & Rosemary Lash & Brow Serum

Rosemary essential oil is known for stimulating hair growth and improving circulation. In combination with castor oil, this serum helps promote lash and brow growth, encouraging healthier and denser hair.

Ingredients:

1 tablespoon castor oil

5 drops rosemary essential oil

Clean mascara wand or dropper bottle

Instructions:

- Mix the castor oil with rosemary essential oil in a small container until well blended.

- Transfer the serum into a clean mascara tube or dropper bottle for easy application.

- For lashes, carefully apply the serum using a clean mascara wand, brushing from the roots of your lashes to the tips. Make sure to cover both the top and bottom lashes.

- For brows, apply with a clean brow brush or use a dropper to place the serum directly on your brows, then massage gently with your fingertips to help the serum absorb.

- Leave the serum on overnight to allow the oils to penetrate the hair follicles and stimulate growth.

- Use the serum every night for at least 4-8 weeks to see noticeable results in lash and brow growth.

118. Castor Oil & Lavender Lash & Brow Serum

Lavender essential oil has soothing properties and helps improve hair health, making it an excellent addition to a growth serum. Castor oil nourishes and moisturizes the follicles, working together to support fuller lashes and brows.

Ingredients:

1 tablespoon castor oil

3 drops lavender essential oil

Clean brow brush or mascara wand

Instructions:

- Combine castor oil and lavender essential oil in a small bowl and mix thoroughly.

- Use a clean mascara wand for lashes or a brow brush for brows to apply the serum.

- For lashes, carefully coat each lash from the root to the tip, being gentle around the delicate eye area.

- For brows, brush the serum onto the brow area, paying attention to areas where the hair is sparse. Gently massage the serum into the skin to stimulate blood flow and help the serum absorb into the follicles.

- Let the serum stay on overnight and wash your face the next morning as part of your routine.

- Use nightly for at least 4-6 weeks to see results in lash and brow thickness.

119. Castor Oil & Jojoba Oil Lash Growth Serum

Jojoba oil mimics the skin's natural oils and helps to moisturize and protect the hair follicles. When paired with castor oil, this serum strengthens lashes and promotes growth, making them appear longer and fuller.

Ingredients:

1 tablespoon castor oil

1 teaspoon jojoba oil

Clean mascara wand or dropper bottle

Instructions:

- In a small bowl, mix castor oil and jojoba oil until fully combined.

- Transfer the serum into a dropper bottle or a clean mascara tube for easy use.

- To apply to your lashes, use a clean mascara wand to gently brush the serum from the roots of your lashes to the tips. Be careful not to use too much product.

- Make sure to coat each lash evenly and avoid getting any oil into your eyes.

- Leave the serum on overnight to allow it to nourish and strengthen the lashes.

- Repeat the process nightly, and expect to see fuller lashes in about 4-8 weeks.

120. Castor Oil & Coconut Oil Brow Growth Serum

Coconut oil is known for its hydrating and nourishing properties, making it ideal for improving the health of your brow hair follicles. Combined with castor oil, this serum helps support eyebrow regrowth, especially in sparse areas.

Ingredients:

1 tablespoon castor oil

1 teaspoon coconut oil

Clean brow brush or dropper bottle

Instructions:

- Melt the coconut oil if solid, then mix it with castor oil in a small bowl until the oils are well blended.

- Use a clean brow brush or dropper to apply the serum to your eyebrows.

- Focus on areas where the brows are thinning or sparse, gently massaging the serum into the brow area to stimulate blood flow and encourage absorption.

- Leave the serum on overnight to let the oils work their magic.

- Use this serum daily for fuller brows and see noticeable results within 4-6 weeks.

121. Castor Oil & Tea Tree Oil Lash & Brow Serum

Tea tree oil is known for its antimicrobial properties, making this serum ideal for cleansing and promoting healthy lash and brow growth. Combined with castor oil, it helps keep hair follicles healthy and free from buildup, encouraging fuller lashes and brows.

Ingredients:

1 tablespoon castor oil

3 drops tea tree essential oil

Clean mascara wand or dropper bottle

Instructions:

- Mix the castor oil and tea tree essential oil in a small container until well combined.

- For lashes, use a clean mascara wand to apply the serum from the roots to the tips. Be cautious to avoid getting the oil in your eyes, as tea tree oil can cause irritation.

- For brows, apply the serum with a brow brush or use your fingertips to massage it gently into the brow area, ensuring it reaches the hair follicles.

- Leave the serum on overnight to promote hair growth and maintain healthy follicles.

- Repeat nightly for best results, and wash your face in the morning.

122. Castor Oil & Argan Oil Lash Growth Serum

Argan oil is rich in fatty acids and vitamin E, making it perfect for nourishing and strengthening hair. Paired with castor oil, this serum boosts lash growth, leaving them longer and healthier over time.

Ingredients:

1 tablespoon castor oil

1 teaspoon argan oil

Clean mascara wand or dropper bottle

Instructions:

- In a small bowl, mix castor oil and argan oil thoroughly.

- Use a clean mascara wand to gently coat your lashes, making sure to apply the serum from the roots to the tips.

- For best results, use a small amount and avoid getting oil into your eyes.

- Leave the serum on overnight to allow the oils to work through the hair follicles and stimulate growth.

- Use the serum nightly for fuller lashes in about 4-8 weeks.

123. Castor Oil & Almond Oil Brow Growth Serum

Almond oil is packed with vitamins that help nourish hair follicles and promote brow growth. When combined with castor oil, this serum helps fill in sparse brows and keep them well-nourished.

Ingredients:

- 1 tablespoon castor oil

- 1 teaspoon almond oil

- Clean brow brush or dropper bottle

Instructions:

- Combine castor oil and almond oil in a small bowl and mix until smooth.

- Use a clean brow brush or dropper to apply the serum to your brows, focusing on areas where the hair is thinner or sparse.

- Massage the serum gently into your brows using your fingertips to stimulate the hair follicles.

- Leave the serum on overnight, allowing the oils to absorb and nourish the brow hair.

- Repeat nightly for fuller brows and store the serum in a small container for easy use.

Make a Difference with Your Review

Help Others Unlock the Power of Castor Oil

"Nature holds the key to our aesthetic, intellectual,cognitive and even spiritual satisfaction." — **E. O. Wilson**

People who give without expectation live longer, happier lives. During our time together, I'd love to do my part in spreading a little of that kindness.

With that in mind, I have a question for you...

Would you help someone you've never met, even if you never got credit for it? Who is this person? They are someone like you—or like you used to be. Maybe they're new to the benefits of natural remedies, wanting healthier skin, stronger hair, or overall wellness, but not quite sure where to start.

At Optilife Publishing, our mission is to make natural health solutions—like castor oil—accessible to everyone. And the only way we can reach more people is by connecting with others who are seeking these solutions.

This is where you come in. Most people judge a book by its cover—and its reviews. So, here's my ask, on behalf of someone out there who's looking for answers: Would you leave a review for this book?

Your review costs nothing, and it takes less than 60 seconds to complete, but it could change someone's life. Your words could help:

- ...One more person discover a natural remedy that improves their skin.

- ...One more individual find a solution for thinning hair.

- ...One more reader benefit from a detox that transforms their health.

If you've found value in this book, your review can guide someone else toward the same transformation. Simply scan the QR code below to leave your review:

If helping someone you've never met brings a smile to your face, then you're the kind of person I'm proud to connect with. Thank you for being a part of this mission!

Now, back to helping you achieve your health goals faster and easier than you ever imagined. There's so much more to share in the coming chapters.

With gratitude,
Optilife Publishing

P.S. - Fun fact: Offering something valuable to others increases your own value. If you know someone who would benefit from the tips in this book, send it their way and spread the knowledge!

Chapter Seven

Body Care (23 Rceipes)

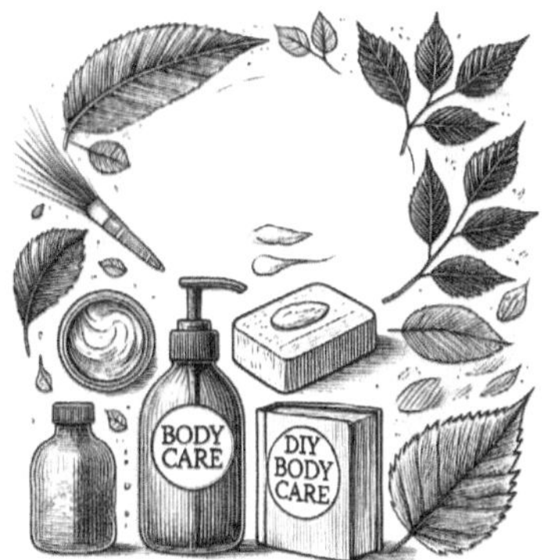

Body Lotions

Castor oil's deep moisturizing abilities make it a perfect base for natural body lotions. Rich in fatty acids, castor oil helps lock in moisture, leaving your skin feeling soft, smooth, and hydrated. In this section, we'll explore a variety of body lotion recipes that blend castor oil with other nourishing ingredients like shea butter, coconut oil, and essential oils to soothe dry skin, improve elasticity, and promote a healthy glow. These lotions are easy to make and provide lasting hydration without the need for harsh chemicals.

124. Castor Oil & Shea Butter Hydrating Body Lotion

This deeply moisturizing body lotion combines the nourishing properties of castor oil and shea butter to keep your skin soft and hydrated. Castor oil penetrates deeply into the skin, while shea butter adds a protective layer to lock in moisture, making this lotion ideal for dry or sensitive skin.

Ingredients:

2 tablespoons castor oil

2 tablespoons shea butter

1 tablespoon coconut oil

10 drops lavender essential oil (optional)

Instructions:

- Melt the shea butter and coconut oil in a double boiler until fully liquefied.

- Remove from heat and stir in castor oil and lavender essential oil.

- Allow the mixture to cool slightly, then transfer to a container and whip it with a hand mixer until it reaches a light, fluffy consistency.

- Apply the lotion to your body after a shower to lock in moisture, and store in a cool, dry place for up to 3 months.

125. Castor Oil & Aloe Vera Soothing Body Lotion

Aloe vera is known for its soothing and healing properties, making it a perfect addition to this body lotion. Combined with castor oil, it provides intense hydration and relief for irritated or sunburned skin, helping to restore your skin's natural balance.

Ingredients:

2 tablespoons castor oil

3 tablespoons aloe vera gel

1 tablespoon coconut oil

5 drops chamomile essential oil (optional)

Instructions:

- In a bowl, mix aloe vera gel and coconut oil until smooth.

- Stir in castor oil and chamomile essential oil for added calming effects.

- Transfer the lotion to a pump bottle for easy use.

- Apply generously to dry or irritated areas to soothe and hydrate the skin. Store in the refrigerator to prolong its shelf life.

126. Castor Oil & Cocoa Butter Nourishing Body Lotion

This rich body lotion combines the nourishing power of castor oil with cocoa butter for a luxurious, deeply hydrating experience. Cocoa butter helps improve skin elasticity and texture, making this lotion perfect for dry skin or stretch marks.

Ingredients:

2 tablespoons castor oil

2 tablespoons cocoa butter

1 tablespoon jojoba oil

10 drops vanilla essential oil (optional)

Instructions:

- Melt cocoa butter in a double boiler, then stir in jojoba oil and castor oil.

- Add vanilla essential oil for a soothing fragrance, if desired.

- Pour the mixture into a container and let it cool until solid, then whip with a hand mixer to create a smooth, creamy texture.

- Use this lotion daily to nourish and soften your skin, particularly on rough areas like elbows and knees.

127. Castor Oil & Rosehip Oil Anti-Aging Body Lotion

Rosehip oil is packed with antioxidants and vitamins A and C, making it a perfect addition to this anti-aging body lotion. Combined with castor oil, this lotion helps reduce the appearance of fine lines and improves skin elasticity, leaving your skin looking youthful and radiant.

Ingredients:

2 tablespoons castor oil

1 tablespoon rosehip oil

1 tablespoon sweet almond oil

10 drops rose essential oil (optional)

Instructions:

- In a small bowl, mix castor oil, rosehip oil, and sweet almond oil until fully blended.

- Add rose essential oil for a light, floral scent, if desired.

- Transfer the lotion to a jar or bottle and apply daily to areas where you want to reduce signs of aging.

- Store the lotion in a cool, dry place and use regularly for firmer, smoother skin.

128. Castor Oil & Honey Body Lotion for Dry Skin

Honey is a natural humectant, meaning it draws moisture into the skin, making it an excellent addition to this hydrating body lotion. When combined with castor oil, this lotion provides long-lasting moisture and helps repair dry, flaky skin.

Ingredients:

2 tablespoons castor oil

1 tablespoon honey

2 tablespoons coconut oil

5 drops lavender essential oil (optional)

Instructions:

- Melt the coconut oil in a double boiler, then stir in honey and castor oil until fully combined.

- Add lavender essential oil to create a calming scent.

- Pour the mixture into a container and allow it to cool.

- Apply the lotion to your body, focusing on particularly dry areas like the elbows, knees, and feet. Store in a cool, dry place.

129. Castor Oil & Avocado Oil Deep Moisture Lotion

Avocado oil is rich in vitamins and fatty acids that nourish and moisturize the skin. When combined with castor oil, this lotion provides intense hydration, making it ideal for very dry or dehydrated skin.

Ingredients:

2 tablespoons castor oil

2 tablespoons avocado oil

1 tablespoon shea butter

5 drops frankincense essential oil (optional)

Instructions:

- Melt the shea butter in a double boiler, then stir in avocado oil and castor oil.

- Add frankincense essential oil for added skin rejuvenation benefits.

- Allow the mixture to cool and transfer it to a jar or container.

- Apply daily to dry skin, particularly in winter months, to maintain hydration and keep your skin soft.

130. Castor Oil & Coconut Oil Refreshing Body Lotion

Coconut oil and castor oil are both excellent moisturizers that penetrate deeply into the skin, leaving it soft and smooth. This lightweight lotion is perfect for everyday use and provides a refreshing, non-greasy hydration that lasts all day.

Ingredients:

2 tablespoons castor oil

2 tablespoons coconut oil

10 drops peppermint essential oil (optional)

Instructions:

- Melt the coconut oil in a double boiler and stir in the castor oil.

- Add peppermint essential oil for a refreshing and cooling sensation.

- Transfer the mixture to a container and let it cool to room temperature.

- Apply after a shower or bath for long-lasting moisture and a refreshing feel. Store in a cool, dry place.

Scrubs

Exfoliation is a key part of maintaining healthy, glowing skin, and castor oil offers a gentle yet effective base for body scrubs. Its emollient properties help soften and hydrate the skin, while natural exfoliants like sugar, salt, or coffee grounds slough away dead skin cells, leaving your skin silky smooth. In this section, we'll delve into a range of castor oil-based scrubs that will exfoliate, nourish, and refresh your skin, making them a perfect addition to your self-care routine.

131. Castor Oil & Sugar Exfoliating Body Scrub

This gentle yet effective sugar scrub combines castor oil's deep moisturizing properties with the exfoliating power of sugar to leave your skin feeling soft and smooth. The sugar crystals help slough off dead skin cells, while castor oil ensures that your skin stays hydrated after exfoliation.

Ingredients:

1/2 cup castor oil

1 cup granulated sugar

10 drops lemon essential oil (optional for a refreshing scent)

Instructions:

- In a bowl, mix the sugar and castor oil until well combined.

- Add the lemon essential oil for a refreshing citrus aroma.

- Use in the shower by applying a handful of the scrub to damp skin, massaging in circular motions to exfoliate.

- Rinse off with warm water and pat your skin dry to reveal soft, smooth skin.

- Store in an airtight container and use 1-2 times a week for best results.

132. Castor Oil & Coffee Ground Revitalizing Scrub

Coffee grounds are known for their invigorating and exfoliating properties. When combined with castor oil, this scrub helps stimulate circulation, reduce the appearance of cellulite, and leave your skin glowing.

Ingredients:

1/2 cup castor oil

1/2 cup used coffee grounds

1 tablespoon coconut oil

Instructions:

- In a bowl, combine the castor oil, coffee grounds, and coconut oil until well mixed.

- Apply the scrub to damp skin, focusing on areas with cellulite or rough patches.

- Massage the scrub in circular motions to exfoliate and stimulate blood flow.

- Rinse off with warm water and follow up with your favorite moisturizer.

- Use this scrub 2-3 times a week to boost circulation and smooth the skin.

133. Castor Oil & Sea Salt Detoxifying Scrub

Sea salt is a natural exfoliant that helps draw out toxins from the skin, while castor oil hydrates and restores moisture balance. This scrub is perfect for detoxifying the skin and improving texture.

Ingredients:

1/2 cup castor oil

1/2 cup sea salt

1 tablespoon olive oil

5 drops eucalyptus essential oil (optional)

Instructions:

- Mix the sea salt, castor oil, and olive oil in a small bowl until well combined.

- Stir in eucalyptus essential oil for a refreshing scent and detoxifying benefits.

- Apply the scrub to wet skin, massaging gently in circular motions to exfoliate.

- Rinse with warm water and follow up with a hydrating lotion.

- Use weekly to detoxify and refresh your skin.

134. Castor Oil & Oatmeal Soothing Scrub

Oatmeal is a gentle exfoliant that helps soothe irritated or sensitive skin, while castor oil provides deep hydration. This scrub is perfect for calming inflamed or dry skin, making it ideal for people with eczema or sensitive skin types.

Ingredients:

1/2 cup castor oil

1/2 cup ground oats

1 tablespoon honey

Instructions:

- Grind the oats into a fine powder using a food processor or blender.

- In a bowl, mix the ground oats, castor oil, and honey until well blended.

- Gently apply the scrub to damp skin, using light, circular motions to exfoliate and soothe.

- Rinse with warm water and pat your skin dry. Follow with a gentle moisturizer for extra hydration.

- Use this scrub 1-2 times a week for soft, calm skin.

135. Castor Oil & Brown Sugar Vanilla Body Scrub

This indulgent scrub combines the exfoliating power of brown sugar with the sweet scent of vanilla. Castor oil helps to hydrate the skin while the sugar exfoliates, leaving your skin feeling soft, smooth, and deliciously scented.

Ingredients:

1/2 cup castor oil

1 cup brown sugar

1 teaspoon vanilla extract

Instructions:

- Mix the brown sugar and castor oil in a bowl until fully combined.

- Add vanilla extract for a sweet, comforting fragrance.

- Apply the scrub to wet skin in the shower, massaging gently to exfoliate and nourish your skin.

- Rinse off with warm water, revealing silky smooth skin.

- Use 2-3 times a week for soft, radiant skin.

136. Castor Oil & Lemon Zest Brightening Scrub

Lemon zest adds a brightening effect to this scrub, which helps to exfoliate and tone the skin. The addition of castor oil ensures your skin stays hydrated and soft after exfoliation, while the citrus adds a refreshing twist.

Ingredients:

1/2 cup castor oil

1 cup granulated sugar

1 tablespoon lemon zest

5 drops lemon essential oil

Instructions:

- Combine the sugar, lemon zest, and castor oil in a bowl until well mixed.

- Stir in the lemon essential oil for extra brightness and a refreshing scent.

- Massage the scrub onto wet skin in circular motions to exfoliate and brighten.

- Rinse thoroughly with warm water, and apply your favorite moisturizer after use.

- Use 1-2 times a week for glowing, even-toned skin.

137. Castor Oil & Baking Soda Gentle Exfoliating Scrub

Baking soda is a gentle exfoliant that helps unclog pores and smooth the skin's surface. Combined with castor oil, this scrub gently exfoliates while hydrating the skin, making it ideal for sensitive or acne-prone skin.

Ingredients:

1/4 cup castor oil

1/4 cup baking soda

1 teaspoon honey

Instructions:

- In a small bowl, mix baking soda, castor oil, and honey until fully blended.

- Apply the scrub to damp skin, gently massaging in circular motions to exfoliate.

- Rinse with warm water and pat dry. Use this scrub 1-2 times a week to maintain clear, smooth skin.

138. Castor Oil & Coconut Sugar Hydrating Scrub

Coconut sugar provides a gentle exfoliation, while castor oil deeply moisturizes the skin. This hydrating scrub is perfect for those looking to exfoliate without stripping the skin of its natural moisture.

Ingredients:

1/2 cup castor oil

1 cup coconut sugar

1 tablespoon coconut oil

Instructions:

- Combine the coconut sugar, castor oil, and coconut oil in a bowl.

- Stir until the ingredients are fully mixed.

- Gently massage the scrub onto damp skin to exfoliate and hydrate.

- Rinse thoroughly with warm water, leaving your skin soft and moisturized.

- Use this scrub 2-3 times a week for soft, smooth skin.

Hand & Foot Treatments

Our hands and feet endure a lot of daily wear and tear, and they often need extra care to keep them soft, smooth, and healthy. Castor oil's thick, nourishing texture makes it an ideal ingredient for treatments targeting cracked heels, rough hands, and cuticle care. This section will explore hand and foot treatments that blend castor oil with healing ingredients like beeswax, aloe vera, and essential oils to restore moisture and repair damaged skin. These treatments are designed to provide intense hydration and relief for dry, rough hands and feet.

139. Castor Oil & Shea Butter Healing Hand Cream

This hand cream combines the intense moisturizing properties of castor oil with the healing power of shea butter. It's perfect for dry, cracked hands, especially in the winter months when skin tends to become more dehydrated. The thick consistency helps to repair damaged skin and keep hands soft and smooth.

Ingredients:

2 tablespoons castor oil

2 tablespoons shea butter

1 tablespoon coconut oil

5 drops lavender essential oil (optional)

Instructions:

- Melt the shea butter and coconut oil in a double boiler until fully liquefied.

- Remove from heat and stir in castor oil and lavender essential oil.

- Allow the mixture to cool slightly, then whip it with a hand mixer until it reaches a creamy consistency.

- Apply generously to your hands, focusing on dry areas. For an overnight treatment, apply the cream and wear cotton gloves to lock in moisture.

- Store in an airtight container and use daily for soft, healed hands.

140. Castor Oil & Peppermint Foot Balm

This foot balm combines castor oil with peppermint essential oil to soothe tired feet and heal cracked heels. Castor oil moisturizes deeply, while peppermint provides a cooling sensation and helps reduce foot odor. Ideal for use after a long day or before bed.

Ingredients:

2 tablespoons castor oil

1 tablespoon beeswax

1 tablespoon coconut oil

10 drops peppermint essential oil

Instructions:

- Melt the beeswax and coconut oil in a double boiler until fully liquefied.

- Stir in the castor oil and peppermint essential oil.

- Pour the mixture into a small jar and let it cool until solid.

- Apply to clean, dry feet, focusing on the heels and any rough patches. For best results, apply the balm before bed and wear socks overnight to lock in moisture.

- Use regularly to keep feet soft and fresh.

141. Castor Oil & Honey Hand Repair Mask

Honey is a natural humectant that helps draw moisture into the skin, making it an excellent addition to this hydrating hand mask. Combined with castor oil, it helps heal and soften rough, dry hands, leaving them silky smooth.

Ingredients:

2 tablespoons castor oil

1 tablespoon honey

1 tablespoon olive oil

Instructions:

- In a small bowl, mix castor oil, honey, and olive oil until well combined.

- Apply a thick layer of the mask to your hands, massaging it into your skin and cuticles.

- Leave the mask on for 15-20 minutes, then rinse with warm water.

- For extra hydration, follow up with a moisturizing hand cream. Use 1-2 times a week for best results.

142. Castor Oil & Epsom Salt Foot Soak

This relaxing foot soak combines the detoxifying effects of Epsom salt with the moisturizing power of castor oil. It's perfect for soothing tired feet, reducing swelling, and softening rough skin, especially after a long day.

Ingredients:

1/4 cup castor oil

1/2 cup Epsom salt

10 drops tea tree essential oil (optional)

Warm water

Instructions:

- Fill a basin or foot spa with warm water.

- Add Epsom salt, castor oil, and tea tree essential oil to the water, stirring to dissolve the salt.

- Soak your feet for 15-20 minutes, allowing the Epsom salt to soothe tired muscles and the castor oil to hydrate your skin.

- After soaking, pat your feet dry and follow with a foot balm or lotion for added moisture.

- Use this foot soak 1-2 times a week to maintain soft, smooth feet.

143. Castor Oil & Beeswax Cuticle Balm

This cuticle balm is perfect for nourishing and moisturizing dry, cracked cuticles. Castor oil helps soften the skin, while beeswax provides a protective barrier that locks in moisture, preventing further dryness or damage.

Ingredients:

2 tablespoons castor oil

1 tablespoon beeswax

1 tablespoon coconut oil

5 drops lavender essential oil (optional)

Instructions:

- Melt the beeswax and coconut oil in a double boiler until fully liquefied.

- Remove from heat and stir in castor oil and lavender essential oil.

- Pour the mixture into a small container and let it cool until solid.

- Apply the balm to your cuticles, massaging it in to soften and nourish the skin.

- Use regularly to keep cuticles hydrated and prevent cracking.

144. Castor Oil & Lemon Foot Scrub for Calluses

This scrub combines castor oil with sugar and lemon to exfoliate rough skin and reduce calluses. The lemon's natural acidity helps soften hard skin, while castor oil keeps your feet hydrated after exfoliation.

Ingredients:

1/4 cup castor oil

1/2 cup granulated sugar

1 tablespoon lemon juice

5 drops lemon essential oil (optional)

Instructions:

- Mix the sugar, lemon juice, and castor oil in a bowl until well combined.

- Use the scrub to massage your feet, focusing on callused areas.

- Rinse with warm water and follow up with a foot balm or lotion to lock in moisture.

- Use this scrub 1-2 times a week to keep your feet soft and smooth.

145. Castor Oil & Avocado Oil Intense Moisturizing Hand Cream

This rich hand cream combines the moisturizing power of castor oil and avocado oil to heal dry, cracked hands. Avocado oil is rich in fatty acids and vitamins, making this cream ideal for deep hydration and repair.

Ingredients:

2 tablespoons castor oil

2 tablespoons avocado oil

1 tablespoon shea butter

5 drops frankincense essential oil (optional)

Instructions:

- Melt the shea butter in a double boiler, then stir in avocado oil and castor oil.

- Remove from heat and allow the mixture to cool slightly before whipping it into a creamy consistency.

- Transfer the cream to a jar and apply generously to your hands, massaging it into the skin.

- Use daily to keep your hands soft and hydrated, especially in dry or cold weather.

146. Castor Oil & Olive Oil Hand & Foot Overnight Treatment

This overnight treatment combines castor oil and olive oil for deep hydration. It's ideal for repairing dry, cracked skin on your hands and feet while you sleep. Olive oil's antioxidants help repair damage, while castor oil locks in moisture.

Ingredients:

- 2 tablespoons castor oil

- 2 tablespoons olive oil

- 5 drops tea tree essential oil (optional)

Instructions:

- Mix castor oil and olive oil in a small bowl until fully combined.

- Massage the oil blend into your hands and feet, focusing on dry or cracked areas.

- For an intensive treatment, wear cotton gloves and socks overnight to help the oils absorb into the skin.

- Wash off any excess oil in the morning and apply a light moisturizer if needed. Use nightly for best results.

Chapter Eight

Massage & Aromatherapy (10 Recipes)

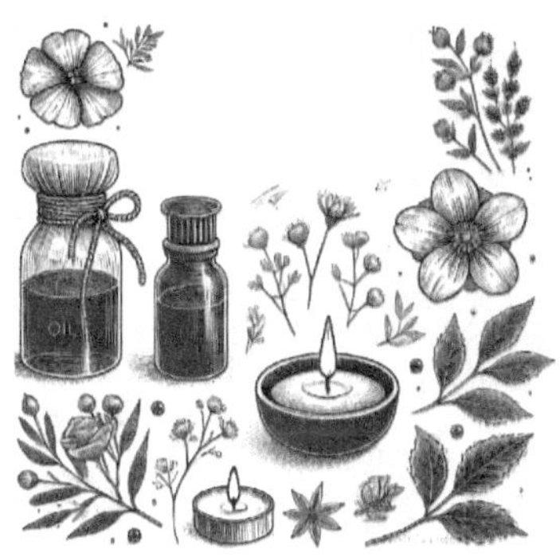

Massage and aromatherapy are ancient practices that promote both physical and mental well-being, offering relaxation and relief from everyday stress. Castor oil's thick, smooth texture makes it an excellent base for massage, as it deeply penetrates the skin to moisturize, reduce inflammation, and relieve tension. When combined with essential oils, castor oil becomes a powerful tool in aromatherapy, enhancing the calming and healing effects of a massage.

In this section, we will explore a variety of **massage oils** and **aromatherapy blends** that harness castor oil's benefits, creating treatments that promote relaxation, improve circulation, ease muscle tension, and support overall wellness. Whether you're looking to unwind after a long day or relieve sore muscles, these recipes will help you incorporate the healing power of castor oil into your self-care routine.

147. Castor Oil & Lavender Relaxation Massage Oil

Lavender is well-known for its calming and relaxing effects, making this massage oil perfect for unwinding after a long day. Castor oil's rich texture helps the oil glide smoothly over the skin, while its moisturizing properties keep the skin hydrated during and after the massage.

Ingredients:

2 tablespoons castor oil

10 drops lavender essential oil

1 tablespoon sweet almond oil

Instructions:

- In a small bowl, mix castor oil, sweet almond oil, and lavender essential oil until well combined.

- Warm the oil slightly by rubbing it between your hands or placing the container in warm water.

- Massage the oil onto your skin in gentle, circular motions, focusing on areas of tension like the shoulders, neck, and lower back.

- Use for full-body relaxation, or focus on problem areas to relieve stress and muscle tension.

148. Castor Oil & Peppermint Muscle Relief Oil

Peppermint essential oil provides a cooling sensation that helps relieve muscle aches and tension. When combined with castor oil, this massage oil is perfect for soothing sore muscles after exercise or a long day.

Ingredients:

2 tablespoons castor oil

10 drops peppermint essential oil

1 tablespoon olive oil

Instructions:

- In a small bowl, mix castor oil, olive oil, and peppermint essential oil.

- Warm the oil slightly before applying to sore muscles, rubbing gently in circular motions.

- Focus on areas of tension, such as the neck, shoulders, and legs, to promote relaxation and relieve discomfort.

- Store the oil in a bottle and use as needed to reduce muscle soreness.

149. Castor Oil & Eucalyptus Invigorating Massage Oil

Eucalyptus oil is known for its refreshing, uplifting aroma, which helps clear the mind and promote better breathing. Combined with castor oil, this invigorating massage oil is great for energizing the body and relieving respiratory congestion.

Ingredients:

2 tablespoons castor oil

10 drops eucalyptus essential oil

1 tablespoon jojoba oil

Instructions:

- In a small bowl, combine castor oil, jojoba oil, and eucalyptus essential oil.

- Warm the oil slightly by placing the container in a bowl of warm water.

- Apply to the chest, shoulders, and back, massaging in long, sweeping motions to promote relaxation and open up the respiratory passages.

- This oil is ideal for use during colds or congestion, or for a refreshing massage to energize the body.

150. Castor Oil & Rosemary Circulation Boost Massage Oil

Rosemary oil is renowned for its ability to improve circulation, making this massage oil perfect for stimulating blood flow. Castor oil enhances the massage's moisturizing effects, making it ideal for those with poor circulation or cold hands and feet.

Ingredients:

2 tablespoons castor oil

10 drops rosemary essential oil

1 tablespoon coconut oil

Instructions:

- In a small bowl, mix castor oil, coconut oil, and rosemary essential oil.

- Warm the oil in your hands or using a bowl of warm water.

- Massage the oil into your skin, focusing on areas like the legs, feet, and hands to promote circulation.

- Use regularly to boost blood flow and reduce cold extremities.

151. Castor Oil & Frankincense Calming Massage Oil

Frankincense has a grounding, calming effect, perfect for meditation or relaxation. When mixed with castor oil, this massage oil offers a luxurious experience that hydrates the skin and eases tension.

Ingredients:

2 tablespoons castor oil

8 drops frankincense essential oil

1 tablespoon grapeseed oil

Instructions:

- Combine castor oil, grapeseed oil, and frankincense essential oil in a small bowl.

- Warm the oil mixture and massage into the skin in long, sweeping strokes.

- Focus on areas of tension to reduce stress, or use during meditation or yoga for a calming experience.

- Store the oil in a small container for regular use.

152. Castor Oil & Chamomile Sleep Massage Oil

Chamomile is well known for its calming, sleep-inducing properties. When combined with castor oil, this massage oil helps relax the body and mind, making it the perfect addition to your bedtime routine.

Ingredients:

2 tablespoons castor oil

8 drops chamomile essential oil

1 tablespoon avocado oil

Instructions:

- In a bowl, mix castor oil, avocado oil, and chamomile essential oil.

- Warm the oil slightly before massaging it onto the body, focusing on areas of stress or tension.

- Use gentle, soothing motions to help the body relax, promoting deeper sleep.

- Use this massage oil as part of your nighttime routine to help ease into restful sleep.

153. Castor Oil & Lemon Uplifting Massage Oil

Lemon essential oil is known for its bright, uplifting properties that promote mental clarity and energize the body. This massage oil, blended with castor oil, is perfect for invigorating the body and refreshing the skin.

Ingredients:

2 tablespoons castor oil

8 drops lemon essential oil

1 tablespoon olive oil

Instructions:

- Combine castor oil, olive oil, and lemon essential oil in a small bowl.

- Warm the oil slightly and apply to the skin using circular massage motions.

- Focus on areas like the back, shoulders, and legs for an energizing massage.

- This oil is ideal for morning use or whenever you need a boost of energy.

154. Castor Oil & Ylang Ylang Sensual Massage Oil

Ylang ylang essential oil is known for its floral, sensual fragrance, making it perfect for a romantic or self-care massage. When mixed with castor oil, it creates a luxurious massage oil that soothes the body and hydrates the skin.

Ingredients:

2 tablespoons castor oil

8 drops ylang ylang essential oil

1 tablespoon jojoba oil

Instructions:

- In a small bowl, mix castor oil, jojoba oil, and ylang ylang essential oil until well combined.

- Warm the oil slightly before massaging it into the skin, using long, gentle strokes.

- Focus on areas of the body that hold tension, allowing the soothing scent of ylang ylang to relax the senses.

- Use for a luxurious, sensual massage experience, whether alone or with a partner.

155. Castor Oil & Ginger Warming Massage Oil

Ginger essential oil has warming properties that make it ideal for relieving sore muscles and improving circulation. Combined with castor oil, this massage oil helps soothe tension and relax tight muscles.

Ingredients:

2 tablespoons castor oil

8 drops ginger essential oil

1 tablespoon coconut oil

Instructions:

- In a small bowl, mix castor oil, coconut oil, and ginger essential oil.

- Warm the oil by rubbing it between your hands or placing it in warm water.

- Apply the oil to sore muscles, massaging deeply to relieve tension and improve circulation.

- Use this oil after exercise or whenever you feel muscle stiffness or soreness.

156. Castor Oil & Clary Sage Balancing Massage Oil

Clary sage is known for its balancing and calming effects, making this massage oil perfect for reducing stress and promoting emotional well-being. Castor oil helps moisturize and nourish the skin while providing a smooth base for massage.

Ingredients:

2 tablespoons castor oil

8 drops clary sage essential oil

1 tablespoon sweet almond oil

Instructions:

- Combine castor oil, sweet almond oil, and clary sage essential oil in a small bowl.

- Warm the mixture slightly and massage onto the skin in long, smooth motions.

- Focus on areas of the body that hold tension, such as the neck and shoulders.

- Use regularly to help balance mood and reduce stress.

Chapter Nine

Baby & Family Care (8 Recipes)

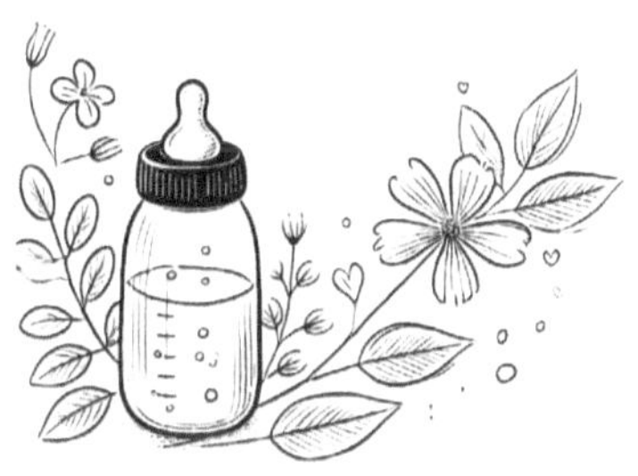

Castor oil's gentle and natural properties make it a safe and effective option for baby and family care. Its moisturizing, healing, and soothing qualities are ideal for addressing common skin concerns, from diaper rash to dry skin, without exposing your family to harsh chemicals. In this section, we'll explore a variety of castor oil-based recipes tailored for the delicate skin of babies and family members, ensuring that everyone benefits from the nurturing effects of natural ingredients.

Gentle Products for Baby Skin

157. Castor Oil & Calendula Diaper Rash Balm

Calendula's soothing and healing properties make it perfect for treating diaper rash. Combined with castor oil, this gentle balm helps reduce inflammation and provides lasting moisture, protecting the baby's delicate skin.

Ingredients:

2 tablespoons castor oil

1 tablespoon calendula-infused olive oil

1 tablespoon beeswax

1 teaspoon shea butter

Instructions:

- Melt the beeswax and shea butter in a double boiler until fully liquefied.

- Stir in castor oil and calendula-infused olive oil, mixing well.

- Pour the mixture into a small jar and allow it to cool until solid.

- Apply a small amount of balm to the baby's clean, dry skin at each diaper change to prevent and soothe diaper rash.

- Store in a cool, dry place and use as needed for protection against irritation.

158. Castor Oil & Coconut Oil Baby Moisturizer

Babies' skin is incredibly delicate and requires gentle hydration. This simple baby moisturizer combines castor oil with coconut oil to provide natural moisture without harsh chemicals, keeping your baby's skin soft and smooth.

Ingredients:

2 tablespoons castor oil

2 tablespoons coconut oil

1 teaspoon aloe vera gel (optional for extra soothing)

Instructions:

- In a small bowl, mix castor oil and coconut oil until fully combined.

- Stir in aloe vera gel for added soothing properties, if desired.

- Gently massage the mixture onto the baby's skin after bath time, focusing on areas prone to dryness.

- Use regularly to keep the baby's skin soft and hydrated. Store in a cool, dry place.

159. Castor Oil & Chamomile Baby Massage Oil

This baby massage oil combines castor oil with the calming effects of chamomile essential oil, perfect for a soothing, bedtime massage. The gentle formula nourishes and protects the baby's delicate skin, helping them relax before sleep.

Ingredients:

2 tablespoons castor oil

1 tablespoon sweet almond oil

3 drops chamomile essential oil

Instructions:

- In a small bowl, mix castor oil and sweet almond oil.

- Add chamomile essential oil and stir gently.

- Warm the oil slightly by rubbing it between your hands and gently massage onto the baby's skin, using soft circular motions.

- Focus on areas like the arms, legs, and back to promote relaxation and bonding.

- Use as part of your baby's bedtime routine to encourage better sleep.

Multipurpose Family Remedies

160. Castor Oil & Aloe Vera Healing Balm

This multipurpose healing balm combines castor oil with aloe vera to provide relief for various skin irritations, including minor cuts, scrapes, and burns. The hydrating and soothing properties of castor oil and aloe vera help speed up healing and prevent scarring.

Ingredients:

2 tablespoons castor oil

2 tablespoons aloe vera gel

1 tablespoon beeswax

5 drops tea tree essential oil (optional for antimicrobial benefits)

Instructions:

- Melt the beeswax in a double boiler until liquefied.

- Stir in castor oil and aloe vera gel, mixing until well combined.

- Add tea tree essential oil for its antibacterial properties, if desired.

- Pour the mixture into a small jar and allow it to cool until solid.

- Apply to minor cuts, scrapes, and burns to soothe and protect the skin. Store in a cool place and use as needed.

161. Castor Oil & Eucalyptus Chest Rub for Colds

This soothing chest rub combines castor oil with eucalyptus essential oil to help relieve congestion and cold symptoms. The warming effect of castor oil paired with eucalyptus helps open the airways and provides comfort during colds.

Ingredients:

2 tablespoons castor oil

1 tablespoon coconut oil

10 drops eucalyptus essential oil

5 drops peppermint essential oil (optional for extra cooling)

Instructions:

- Melt the coconut oil in a double boiler until liquefied, then stir in castor oil.

- Add eucalyptus and peppermint essential oils, mixing well.

- Pour the mixture into a small jar and let it cool until solid.

- Rub a small amount onto the chest and throat to help clear congestion and soothe the symptoms of colds. Use as needed, especially before bedtime.

162. Castor Oil & Clove Toothache Relief

Clove oil is known for its pain-relieving properties, making it perfect for treating toothaches. Combined with castor oil, this remedy provides relief for sore gums and toothaches, while helping reduce inflammation.

Ingredients:

1 tablespoon castor oil

5 drops clove essential oil

Instructions:

- In a small bowl, mix castor oil and clove essential oil until well combined.

- Using a clean cotton swab, apply the mixture directly to the sore tooth or gums.

- Repeat as needed to relieve pain and discomfort. This remedy is best used for temporary relief before seeking professional dental care.

163. Castor Oil & Lavender Sleep Aid Balm

This soothing balm uses the calming effects of lavender essential oil along with the moisturizing properties of castor oil to help promote relaxation and restful sleep. Ideal for rubbing onto pulse points or the soles of the feet before bedtime.

Ingredients:

2 tablespoons castor oil

1 tablespoon beeswax

10 drops lavender essential oil

Instructions:

- Melt the beeswax in a double boiler until fully liquefied.

- Stir in castor oil and lavender essential oil, mixing until well combined.

- Pour the mixture into a small jar and allow it to cool until solid.

- Apply a small amount to pulse points (wrists, neck) or the soles of your feet before bed to promote a restful night's sleep.

164. Castor Oil & Arnica Bruise Soothing Balm

Arnica is known for its ability to reduce bruising and swelling. Combined with castor oil, this balm helps to soothe bruised skin and reduce discoloration and swelling, speeding up the healing process.

Ingredients:

2 tablespoons castor oil

1 tablespoon arnica-infused oil

1 tablespoon beeswax

Instructions:

- Melt the beeswax in a double boiler until liquefied.

- Stir in castor oil and arnica-infused oil, mixing until well blended.

- Pour the mixture into a small jar and allow it to cool until solid.

- Apply to bruised or swollen areas 2-3 times a day to reduce inflammation and discoloration.

Chapter Ten

Home Remedies (15 Recipes)

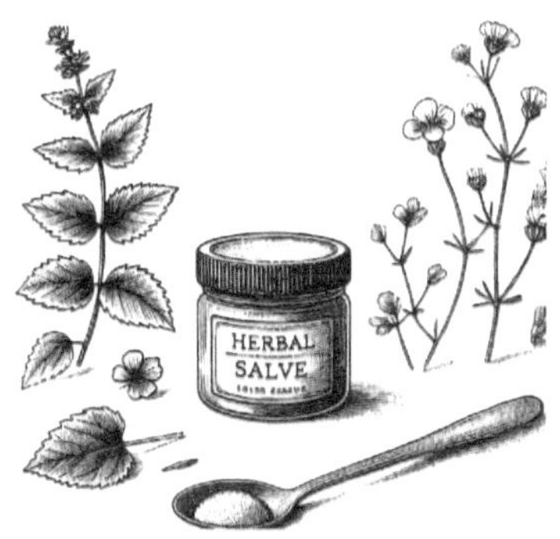

Castor oil's versatile healing properties extend beyond skincare to address a variety of common household ailments. In this section, we'll explore **Home Remedies** that leverage the natural power of castor oil to provide relief for colds, digestive issues, and minor first aid needs. These remedies are designed to offer gentle, effective solutions without the need for harsh chemicals or synthetic ingredients, making them a great choice for families seeking natural alternatives.

Cold Relief

165. Castor Oil & Eucalyptus Vapor Rub

This vapor rub uses the decongestant properties of eucalyptus essential oil combined with the moisturizing effects of castor oil to provide relief from cold symptoms. The rub helps to clear the airways and ease breathing, making it especially useful for nighttime congestion.

Ingredients:

2 tablespoons castor oil

1 tablespoon coconut oil

10 drops eucalyptus essential oil

5 drops peppermint essential oil (optional for extra cooling)

Instructions:

- Melt the coconut oil in a double boiler until liquefied, then stir in castor oil.

- Add eucalyptus and peppermint essential oils, mixing well.

- Pour the mixture into a small jar and let it cool until solid.

- Rub a small amount onto the chest, throat, and upper back to help clear airways and ease breathing during colds. Use as needed, particularly before bedtime.

166. Castor Oil & Ginger Warming Compress

Ginger's warming properties, combined with castor oil, create a compress that helps relieve chest congestion and promotes circulation, making it perfect for soothing cold symptoms and easing respiratory discomfort.

Ingredients:

2 tablespoons castor oil

1 tablespoon ginger juice (freshly grated ginger)

A warm, damp cloth

Instructions:

- Mix castor oil with freshly squeezed ginger juice in a small bowl.

- Warm the mixture slightly, being careful not to overheat.

- Apply the mixture to the chest and cover with a warm, damp cloth.

- Leave the compress on for 15-20 minutes to relieve chest conges-tion. Use 1-2 times a day during colds to promote easier breathing and reduce congestion.

167. Castor Oil & Lemon Steam Inhalation

Steam inhalation helps open the nasal passages and soothe respiratory discomfort. Adding castor oil and lemon essential oil to the steam pro-vides moisturizing and cleansing effects, helping to reduce congestion and refresh the airways.

Ingredients:

1 tablespoon castor oil

5 drops lemon essential oil

A bowl of hot water

A towel

Instructions:

- Add castor oil and lemon essential oil to a bowl of hot water.

- Place your face over the bowl and drape a towel over your head to trap the steam.

- Inhale deeply for 10-15 minutes, allowing the steam to clear your sinuses and reduce congestion.

- Repeat 1-2 times a day during cold symptoms for relief.

168. Castor Oil & Turmeric Immune-Boosting Tea

This soothing tea combines the anti-inflammatory properties of turmeric with castor oil to help strengthen the immune system and reduce inflammation during colds. The warming drink can also soothe sore throats and support overall recovery.

Ingredients:

1/2 teaspoon castor oil

1/2 teaspoon ground turmeric

1 teaspoon honey

1 cup warm water or herbal tea

Instructions:

- In a cup of warm water or herbal tea, mix castor oil, turmeric, and honey until fully dissolved.

- Drink the tea slowly, allowing the warmth to soothe your throat and boost your immune system.

- Enjoy once daily during colds to promote faster recovery and reduce inflammation.

169. Castor Oil & Peppermint Foot Soak for Fever Relief

This foot soak combines the cooling properties of peppermint with the moisturizing benefits of castor oil to help reduce fever and promote relaxation during colds. It's especially useful when you need to cool down and soothe achy muscles.

Ingredients:

2 tablespoons castor oil

10 drops peppermint essential oil

Warm water (enough to fill a foot basin)

Instructions:

- Fill a foot basin with warm water and add castor oil and peppermint essential oil.

- Soak your feet for 15-20 minutes, allowing the cooling sensation of the peppermint and the moisturizing effect of castor oil to relax your body and reduce fever.

- Use as needed during colds to promote relaxation and bring down body temperature.

Digestive Aids

170. Castor Oil Digestive Tonic for Constipation

Castor oil has long been valued as a natural remedy for constipation due to its gentle yet effective laxative properties. This digestive tonic provides quick relief by stimulating bowel movements and improving digestion. It's a simple, natural solution for occasional constipation, helping you stay regular without relying on harsh synthetic laxatives.

Ingredients:

1 teaspoon castor oil

1 cup warm water or herbal tea

1 teaspoon lemon juice (optional for taste)

Instructions:

- In a cup of warm water or herbal tea, stir in the castor oil and lemon juice. Ensure that the mixture is well-blended for even intake.

- Drink the tonic slowly on an empty stomach, preferably in the morning to allow time for digestion to occur during the day.

- Expect results within 4-6 hours. It's important to stay hydrated after drinking the tonic to aid the body's natural detoxification process.

- Use this remedy occasionally to relieve constipation, but avoid frequent use to prevent dependency on laxatives. If symptoms persist, consult a healthcare professional.

171. Castor Oil & Ginger Bloating Relief

Ginger is well known for its anti-inflammatory and digestive benefits, particularly for reducing bloating, gas, and discomfort. Paired with castor oil, this remedy offers soothing relief from digestive discomfort, while supporting healthy digestion and easing feelings of heaviness after meals.

Ingredients:

1 teaspoon castor oil

1/2 teaspoon grated fresh ginger or 1/4 teaspoon ground ginger

1 cup warm water

Instructions:

- In a cup of warm water, mix the castor oil and fresh or ground ginger. Stir thoroughly until the ginger dissolves, creating a smooth mixture.

- Drink the mixture slowly to allow the active ingredients to settle and begin relieving digestive discomfort.

- For best results, consume this remedy after meals to promote digestion and ease bloating or gas.

- You can also take this remedy as needed when experiencing digestive discomfort, but it's gentle enough for regular use after larger meals.

172. Castor Oil Abdominal Massage for Digestive Relief

Massaging castor oil onto the abdomen helps stimulate digestion, relieve constipation, and reduce bloating by improving circulation and encouraging the natural movement of the digestive system. This method provides a soothing, non-invasive way to relieve digestive discomfort while nurturing gut health.

Ingredients:

1 tablespoon castor oil

A warm cloth

Instructions:

- Warm the castor oil slightly by rubbing it between your palms or placing it in a bowl of warm water. This helps the oil penetrate the skin more effectively.

- Apply the warm oil to your abdomen, starting just below your ribs and using gentle, circular motions.

- Continue the massage for 5-10 minutes, focusing on areas around the navel and moving in a clockwise direction, which follows the natural flow of digestion.

- After the massage, cover your abdomen with a warm cloth for another 10-15 minutes to encourage absorption and stimulate digestion.

- Repeat as needed to support digestion and relieve discomfort, especially before bed or in the morning.

173. Castor Oil & Peppermint Digestive Soother

Peppermint is highly regarded for its ability to calm the digestive system and relieve symptoms of indigestion, nausea, and bloating. When paired with castor oil, this remedy provides quick, soothing relief for digestive upset, helping you feel more comfortable after meals.

Ingredients:

1 teaspoon castor oil

5 drops peppermint essential oil

1 cup warm water

Instructions:

- Mix castor oil and peppermint essential oil in a cup of warm water, stirring until the oil is evenly distributed.

- Sip the mixture slowly, allowing the peppermint to soothe the digestive system and castor oil to promote gentle relief.

- Use this remedy after meals or when experiencing symptoms of indigestion, bloating, or nausea. If needed, you can increase the peppermint oil to 6-7 drops for more intense relief.

- For best results, avoid drinking large amounts of cold water during meals, as this can exacerbate indigestion.

174. Castor Oil & Fennel Seeds Digestive Tea

Fennel seeds are a well-known remedy for relieving gas and bloating, while castor oil helps promote smoother digestion. This gentle tea provides a comforting way to alleviate digestive issues and support overall gut health, especially after large meals.

Ingredients:

1/2 teaspoon castor oil

1 teaspoon fennel seeds

1 cup boiling water

Honey (optional for taste)

Instructions:

- Steep the fennel seeds in boiling water for 5-10 minutes to release their digestive-supporting oils.

- Strain the tea into a cup and stir in the castor oil until it dissolves completely.

- Add honey to taste, if desired, for a hint of sweetness.

- Sip the tea slowly to relieve gas, bloating, and indigestion. You can drink this tea after meals or when digestive discomfort occurs.

- For best results, use this tea 1-2 times a day to promote healthy digestion and prevent bloating, especially after larger or heavier meals.

Simple First Aid Solutions

175. Castor Oil & Honey Wound Healing Balm

Castor oil's moisturizing and anti-inflammatory properties make it ideal for wound healing, while honey is known for its antibacterial effects. This balm can be applied to minor cuts, scrapes, and abrasions to promote healing and prevent infection.

Ingredients:

2 tablespoons castor oil

1 tablespoon raw honey

1 teaspoon beeswax

Instructions:

- Melt the beeswax in a double boiler until fully liquefied, then remove from heat.

- Stir in the castor oil and honey, mixing well to combine the ingredients.

- Pour the mixture into a small jar and allow it to cool until solid.

- Apply a small amount of the balm to clean, dry wounds, cuts, or abrasions. Reapply 1-2 times a day to promote healing and keep the area moisturized.

- Store in a cool, dry place and use as needed.

176. Castor Oil & Lavender Burn Relief Gel

Lavender essential oil has natural pain-relieving and antiseptic properties, making it ideal for soothing minor burns. Castor oil helps keep the skin moisturized and aids in healing by preventing dryness and cracking.

Ingredients:

2 tablespoons castor oil

1 tablespoon aloe vera gel

10 drops lavender essential oil

Instructions:

- In a small bowl, combine castor oil, aloe vera gel, and lavender essential oil until smooth.

- Gently apply the gel to the affected area, taking care not to rub too hard on sensitive skin.

- Reapply the gel as needed to keep the burn moisturized and reduce pain.

- Use this remedy for minor burns and sunburns, but seek medical attention for severe burns. Store in a cool place, and apply several times daily for best results.

177. Castor Oil & Tea Tree Insect Bite Soother

Tea tree oil is a powerful natural antiseptic, while castor oil soothes the itch and reduces inflammation. This remedy helps to relieve itching and swelling from insect bites, while also preventing infection.

Ingredients:

1 tablespoon castor oil

5 drops tea tree essential oil

Instructions:

- Mix castor oil and tea tree essential oil in a small bowl until fully blended.

- Use a clean cotton swab to apply the mixture directly to insect bites, gently dabbing the area.

- Reapply the mixture 2-3 times a day to relieve itching and reduce swelling.

- Use this remedy for mosquito bites, bee stings, and other minor insect irritations. Avoid scratching the bites to prevent infection.

178. Castor Oil & Arnica Bruise Reducing Ointment

Arnica is well known for its ability to reduce bruising and inflammation. When combined with castor oil, this ointment helps to heal bruises faster by reducing discoloration and swelling, making it perfect for minor bumps and contusions.

Ingredients:

2 tablespoons castor oil

1 tablespoon arnica-infused oil

1 teaspoon beeswax

Instructions:

- Melt the beeswax in a double boiler until fully liquefied.

- Stir in the castor oil and arnica-infused oil, blending the ingredients thoroughly.

- Pour the mixture into a small jar and let it cool to form a solid ointment.

- Gently massage the ointment onto bruised areas 2-3 times a day to reduce swelling and discoloration.

- Use regularly for faster healing and relief from bruising. Store in a cool, dry place.

179. Castor Oil & Calendula First Aid Salve

Calendula is known for its gentle healing properties, making it perfect for a multipurpose first aid salve. Combined with castor oil, this salve helps treat minor cuts, scrapes, and skin irritations, speeding up healing and preventing dryness.

Ingredients:

2 tablespoons castor oil

1 tablespoon calendula-infused olive oil

1 teaspoon beeswax

Instructions:

- Melt the beeswax in a double boiler until liquefied.

- Stir in castor oil and calendula-infused olive oil, blending until smooth.

- Pour the mixture into a small jar and allow it to cool until it solidifies.

- Apply the salve to cuts, scrapes, and irritated skin 1-2 times a day to promote healing and keep the skin moisturized.

- Use this remedy as a multipurpose salve for family first aid needs. Store in a cool, dry place.

Chapter Eleven

Household & Cleaning (10 Recipes)

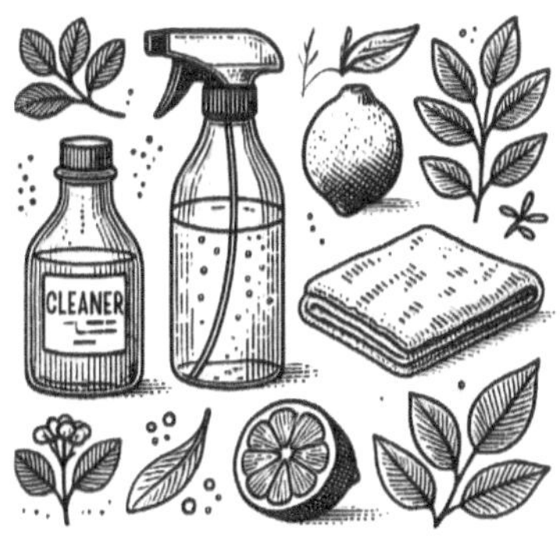

Castor oil isn't just for skincare or health remedies—it can also be an essential ingredient in creating natural, eco-friendly solutions for home care. From polishing furniture to creating gentle but effective cleaning agents, castor oil helps you maintain a clean and healthy environment without resorting to harsh chemicals. In this section, we'll explore versatile cleaning solutions and polishes that protect and shine your home while keeping it toxin-free.

Cleaning Solutions

180. Castor Oil & Lemon All-Purpose Cleaner

This all-purpose cleaner combines castor oil with the antibacterial and freshening power of lemon essential oil, creating an effective solution for cleaning surfaces around your home. It works well on countertops, sinks, and other hard surfaces, leaving a clean, fresh scent behind.

Ingredients:

1/4 cup castor oil

1/2 cup white vinegar

10 drops lemon essential oil

1 cup water

Spray bottle

Instructions:

- In a spray bottle, combine castor oil, white vinegar, and water. Shake well to mix the ingredients.

- Add the lemon essential oil and shake again to combine.

- Spray the cleaner onto surfaces like countertops, kitchen appliances, and bathroom sinks. Wipe with a clean cloth or sponge.

- Store in a cool place and shake before each use, as the ingredients may separate over time.

181. Castor Oil & Baking Soda Scrub

This simple scrub combines castor oil with baking soda to create a powerful, natural cleaner that's perfect for scrubbing sinks, bathtubs, and tough stains. The gentle abrasiveness of baking soda works well with castor oil's moisturizing properties, leaving surfaces clean without scratching.

Ingredients:

2 tablespoons castor oil

1/4 cup baking soda

5 drops tea tree essential oil (optional for antibacterial properties)

Instructions:

- In a bowl, mix the castor oil and baking soda to form a thick paste.

- Add tea tree essential oil if you prefer extra antibacterial protection.

- Use a cloth or sponge to apply the scrub to dirty surfaces like sinks, bathtubs, or stovetops. Scrub in circular motions to lift grime and stains.

- Rinse with warm water and wipe dry. Store any leftover scrub in a small jar for future use.

182. Castor Oil & Vinegar Glass Cleaner

For streak-free glass and mirrors, this natural glass cleaner uses the combination of castor oil and vinegar. Castor oil breaks down smudges and dirt, while vinegar leaves a streak-free shine. This is a great eco-friendly alternative to commercial glass cleaners.

Ingredients:

1 tablespoon castor oil

1/4 cup white vinegar

1 cup water

10 drops peppermint essential oil (optional for a fresh scent)

Spray bottle

Instructions:

- In a spray bottle, combine castor oil, white vinegar, and water. Shake well to mix.

- Add peppermint essential oil for a refreshing scent, then shake the bottle again.

- Spray onto glass surfaces, mirrors, or windows, and wipe clean with a microfiber cloth or newspaper for a streak-free finish.

- Shake the bottle before each use, as the oil may separate over time.

183. Castor Oil & Lavender Floor Cleaner

This floor cleaner is gentle on hardwood, tile, and laminate floors, using castor oil to provide a natural shine without leaving behind harmful residues. The addition of lavender essential oil helps disinfect while leaving a calming aroma throughout your home.

Ingredients:

1/4 cup castor oil

1/2 cup white vinegar

10 drops lavender essential oil

1 gallon warm water

Instructions:

- In a large bucket, mix castor oil, white vinegar, and warm water.

- Stir in lavender essential oil for its antibacterial properties and soothing scent.

- Mop your floors as usual, using the solution to clean and shine surfaces. Avoid using too much liquid on hardwood floors to prevent warping.

- Allow the floors to air dry for a clean, natural shine.

184. Castor Oil & Citrus Degreaser

This degreaser is excellent for cutting through tough grease and grime on stovetops, ovens, and kitchen surfaces. Castor oil helps lift the grease, while citrus essential oil breaks it down, leaving your kitchen sparkling clean.

Ingredients:

2 tablespoons castor oil

1/4 cup white vinegar

10 drops orange essential oil

1 cup water

Spray bottle

Instructions:

- In a spray bottle, combine castor oil, white vinegar, and water. Shake to mix the ingredients.

- Add orange essential oil, known for its powerful degreasing properties, and shake again.

- Spray the mixture onto greasy surfaces, like stovetops or oven doors, and let it sit for 5-10 minutes.

- Wipe away the grease with a cloth or sponge. For tough spots, scrub lightly to lift the grime. Shake before each use.

Polishes for Eco-Friendly Home Care

185. Castor Oil & Beeswax Wood Furniture Polish

This natural wood polish combines the moisturizing properties of castor oil with the protective benefits of beeswax, leaving wooden surfaces with a rich, shiny finish. It not only restores the wood's natural beauty but also protects it from wear and tear.

Ingredients:

2 tablespoons castor oil

1 tablespoon beeswax

5 drops lemon essential oil (optional for a fresh scent)

Instructions:

- Melt the beeswax in a double boiler until fully liquefied.

- Stir in castor oil and lemon essential oil, mixing thoroughly.

- Pour the mixture into a small jar and allow it to cool and solidify.

- To use, scoop a small amount of the polish onto a soft cloth and rub it into wooden furniture in circular motions. Buff with a clean cloth to enhance the shine.

- Use regularly to maintain wood's natural luster and protect it from drying out.

186. Castor Oil & Vinegar Stainless Steel Polish

Stainless steel surfaces can lose their shine over time. This natural polish uses castor oil and vinegar to clean and restore the sparkle to stainless steel appliances, sinks, and fixtures, without leaving streaks or residue.

Ingredients:

1 tablespoon castor oil

1/4 cup white vinegar

1 cup water

5 drops tea tree essential oil (optional for extra shine)

Spray bottle

Instructions:

- Combine castor oil, vinegar, and water in a spray bottle and shake well.

- Add tea tree essential oil for its antibacterial properties and a fresh finish.

- Spray the mixture onto stainless steel surfaces and wipe clean with a microfiber cloth to avoid streaks.

- Buff with a dry cloth for a shiny, streak-free finish.

187. Castor Oil & Olive Oil Leather Conditioner

Leather furniture and accessories can dry out and crack without proper care. This conditioner uses castor oil and olive oil to moisturize and protect leather, restoring its natural softness and shine while keeping it supple.

Ingredients:

1 tablespoon castor oil

1 tablespoon olive oil

5 drops lemon essential oil (optional for fragrance)

Instructions:

- Mix castor oil and olive oil in a small bowl until fully blended.

- Add lemon essential oil for a light, refreshing scent.

- Apply a small amount of the mixture to a soft cloth and gently rub it into leather furniture, bags, or shoes in circular motions.

- Let the conditioner sit for 10-15 minutes, then buff the surface with a clean cloth to remove excess oil and restore the leather's shine.

- Use this conditioner regularly to maintain leather's natural moisture and prevent cracking.

188. Castor Oil & Citrus Brass Polish

Brass surfaces can tarnish over time, losing their shine. This polish uses castor oil and citrus essential oil to gently clean and restore brass's natural luster without the use of harsh chemicals.

Ingredients:

1 tablespoon castor oil

1 tablespoon baking soda

10 drops lemon or orange essential oil

Instructions:

- In a small bowl, mix castor oil, baking soda, and citrus essential oil to form a paste.

- Apply the paste to brass items using a soft cloth or sponge, rubbing gently to remove tarnish.

- Rinse the brass with warm water and buff dry with a clean cloth for a polished finish.

- Repeat as needed to maintain brass's bright shine.

189. Castor Oil & Beeswax Car Dashboard Polish

This dashboard polish helps restore shine to car interiors while providing a protective layer to keep the dashboard from cracking under the sun's rays. Castor oil nourishes the material, while beeswax adds a lasting shine.

Ingredients:

2 tablespoons castor oil

1 tablespoon beeswax

5 drops lavender essential oil (optional for a pleasant scent)

Instructions:

- Melt the beeswax in a double boiler until liquefied.

- Stir in castor oil and lavender essential oil, mixing well.

- Pour the mixture into a small jar and let it cool until solid.

- To use, apply a small amount of the polish to a soft cloth and gently rub it onto the car dashboard, focusing on dry or faded areas.

- Buff with a clean cloth to restore shine and leave a protective coating. Repeat every few months to maintain the dashboard's condition.

Chapter Twelve

Myths and Facts About Castor Oil

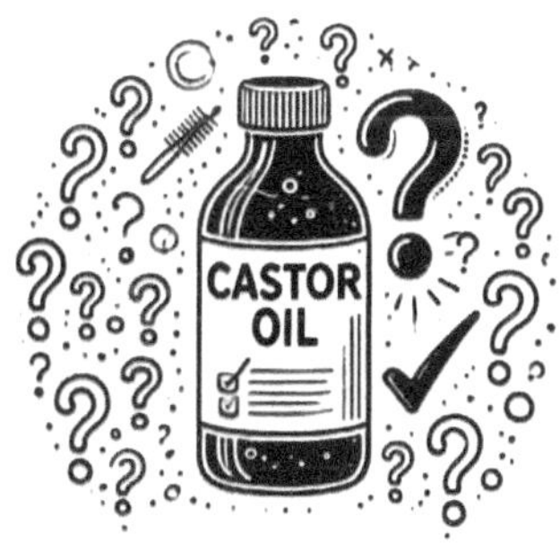

Castor oil has been used for centuries across various cultures, prized for its wide range of applications, from medicinal to cosmetic and industrial uses. However, like many natural remedies, castor oil is surrounded by myths and misconceptions, often making it difficult to separate fact from fiction. In this section, we'll explore common myths, evidence-based facts, and address concerns about castor oil to help readers understand its true benefits and limitations.

Common Misconceptions About Castor Oil

"Castor Oil is a Quick Fix for Hair Growth" One of the most popular misconceptions is that castor oil will dramatically increase hair growth overnight. This belief has been fueled by social media and anecdotal reports claiming rapid results after just a few applications. However, the reality is more nuanced. Castor oil contains ricinoleic acid, which has moisturizing and anti-inflammatory properties, but it doesn't speed up the natural hair growth cycle. Castor oil can improve the overall condition of your hair by strengthening it and reducing breakage, which might give the appearance of faster growth. Regular use can enhance shine, prevent split ends, and keep the scalp hydrated, but it will not make hair grow noticeably faster in a short time.

"Castor Oil Can Cure Skin Conditions Like Acne or Psoriasis" Many people believe castor oil is a miracle solution for curing skin conditions such as acne, psoriasis, or eczema. While it does have anti-inflammatory and antimicrobial properties, these are not strong enough to single-handedly cure chronic skin disorders. Overusing castor oil on sensitive or acne-prone skin may even clog pores, leading to further irritation. Castor oil can help soothe irritated skin, thanks to its moisturizing properties, and may support the healing process of minor skin issues. However, for chronic conditions like acne or psoriasis, castor oil should be seen as a supplementary treatment rather than a cure. Dermatologist-prescribed treatments are often necessary for significant results.

"Castor Oil is Unsafe Because it Comes from the Ricin Plant" Another common misconception is that castor oil is unsafe for use because it is derived from the castor bean plant, which contains ricin—a potent toxin. This fear has led some people to avoid castor oil altogether, despite its widespread use in both traditional medicine and modern beauty products. While the raw castor bean does contain ricin, the extraction and processing of castor oil remove this toxic substance completely. Castor oil sold for medicinal, cosmetic, and industrial use is thoroughly purified and is safe for both topical application and ingestion in recommended amounts. There is no risk of ricin poisoning from properly processed castor oil.

"Castor Oil Can Induce Labor in Pregnant Women Anytime" Castor oil has been traditionally used to induce labor in overdue pregnancies, which has created the misconception that it is dangerous for pregnant women at any stage. Some people believe that any form of castor oil use, even topical, could trigger early labor. Castor oil can indeed stimulate uterine contractions if taken orally in significant amounts. However, using castor oil topically or in small quantities for skin or hair care during pregnancy is generally safe and will not induce labor. Pregnant women should avoid ingesting castor oil without medical supervision, especially before full-term pregnancy, as it can cause unpleasant side effects like nausea or diarrhea.

"Castor Oil Works Instantly as a Laxative" Many people assume that castor oil will provide immediate relief from constipation due to its well-known laxative properties. This leads to the misconception that castor oil is an instant remedy for digestive discomfort. While castor oil is an effective stimulant laxative, it does not work immediately. It usually takes 4-6 hours to induce a bowel movement after ingestion. Moreover, castor oil should be used sparingly for constipation relief, as overuse can lead to dehydration and dependency. Always follow proper dosage guidelines and consult with a healthcare professional for regular digestive issues.

"Castor Oil is Hypoallergenic and Safe for Everyone" It's a common belief that because castor oil is a natural product, it is hypoallergenic and completely safe for all skin types, including those with sensitive skin or allergies. While castor oil is relatively gentle, it can still cause adverse reactions in some individuals. Like any oil or cosmetic product, castor oil can cause allergic reactions, particularly in people with sensitive skin.

Before using it extensively, it's wise to perform a patch test to check for any redness, irritation, or itching. If a reaction occurs, discontinue use and seek alternatives.

Evidence-Based Facts About Castor Oil

1. Castor Oil's Laxative Properties

Castor oil's use as a natural laxative is backed by both historical practice and modern research. The active ingredient, ricinoleic acid, stimulates peristalsis, the contractions of the intestines, promoting bowel movements. This is why castor oil has been widely used for relieving occasional constipation.

Study: A 2011 study published in *Complementary Therapies in Clinical Practice* examined the effects of castor oil packs on elderly patients in nursing homes suffering from chronic constipation. The study found that while the oil did not significantly increase the frequency of bowel movements, it did improve the patient's subjective experience by reducing discomfort and straining associated with bowel movements. The packs helped alleviate the sensation of incomplete evacuation, suggesting castor oil's utility in managing constipation . Another clinical study confirmed castor oil's effectiveness in stimulating complete bowel evacuation before medical procedures, reinforcing its role as a stimulant laxative in controlled dosages.

Safety Note: Castor oil should be used sparingly for constipation relief, as overuse can lead to dehydration and dependence on laxatives. It is recommended to use it under medical supervision, especially for prolonged or chronic cases.

2. Anti-inflammatory and Antimicrobial Properties

Ricinoleic acid, which makes up almost 90% of castor oil, is responsible for the oil's significant anti-inflammatory effects. These properties make castor oil useful in reducing swelling and inflammation, whether applied to the skin for conditions like dermatitis or used to soothe minor wounds and irritations. Furthermore, its antimicrobial effects provide an added layer of protection against infections.

Study: Research published in *Planta Medica* in 2000 demonstrated that ricinoleic acid significantly reduced inflammation in animal models, particularly reducing paw edema in rats, which is an indication of its anti-inflammatory potential. The same study found that ricinoleic acid's effects were comparable to capsaicin in reducing pain and inflammation but without the irritation often associated with capsaicin

Natural Remedy Ideas. Additionally, castor oil has shown antibacterial and antifungal properties, making it a valuable natural remedy for minor infections and wounds.

This dual-action (anti-inflammatory and antimicrobial) makes castor oil a popular choice for topical skin treatments, where it can soothe irritation and prevent infection in one step.

3. Castor Oil for Joint and Muscle Pain

Castor oil is frequently used to alleviate joint and muscle pain, largely due to the anti-inflammatory effects of ricinoleic acid. This fatty acid penetrates the skin and reduces inflammation and swelling in joints and tissues, providing relief from conditions like arthritis, sore muscles, and even minor injuries.

Study: A comparative study published in *Phytotherapy Research* found that castor oil was as effective as the nonsteroidal anti-inflammatory drug (NSAID) diclofenac in treating knee osteoarthritis. The patients who received castor oil capsules reported similar pain relief and reduction in inflammation as those treated with diclofenac, but with fewer gastrointestinal side effects . This suggests that castor oil could be a viable natural alternative or complementary treatment for joint and muscle pain, particularly for individuals looking to avoid the adverse effects associated with long-term NSAID use.

Chapter Thirteen

Ethical Sourcing and Sustainability of Castor Oil

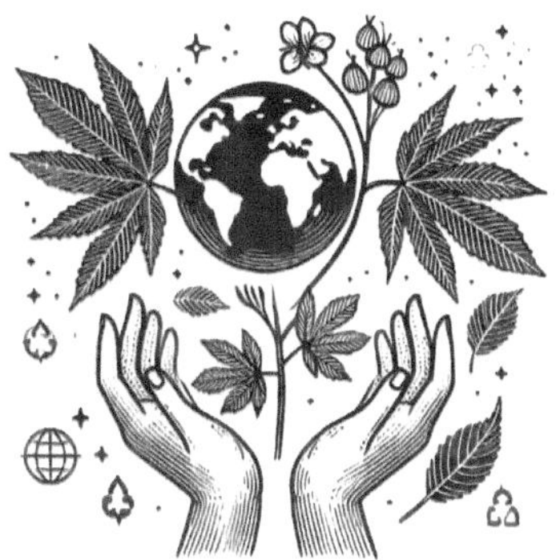

As the demand for castor oil increases in industries such as cosmetics, pharmaceuticals, and biofuels, it is important to ensure that its production aligns with ethical and sustainable practices. This section covers the key areas related to the sourcing and sustainability of castor oil, from farming practices to the broader environmental and social impacts.

Ethical production begins with how castor beans are cultivated. Many castor farms are located in developing regions such as India, which produces the majority of the world's supply. Ethical production focuses on ensuring fair labor practices, safe working conditions, and proper wages for farmers. This includes avoiding child labor and ensuring that farming communities benefit economically from the cultivation of castor beans. Certified organic and fair trade practices are becoming more prevalent, allowing consumers to choose products that support ethical labor conditions and environmentally friendly farming practices.

Sustainability in castor oil production extends beyond human labor to the environmental footprint of farming. Castor plants themselves are relatively drought-resistant and can grow in semi-arid regions with minimal need for irrigation or fertilizers. This makes them more sustainable compared to other oil crops that demand intensive water and chemical inputs. However, large-scale production can still lead to soil depletion and biodiversity loss if not managed carefully. Sustainable farming practices include crop rotation, organic farming methods, and the prevention of deforestation. As castor oil increasingly becomes a feedstock for biofuel production, the environmental benefits are magnified. Its use in bioplastics and biofuels reduces reliance on fossil fuels, contributing to a reduction in carbon emissions. However, ensuring that castor farming does not lead to monocultures or negatively impact local ecosystems is critical to maintaining its sustainability.

For sustainability to thrive, consumer awareness is essential. Consumers play a vital role in driving the demand for ethically sourced and environmentally responsible castor oil. Brands that commit to transparency in their supply chains and clearly label products with fair trade or organic certifications help consumers make informed choices. As awareness grows, more companies are opting for certified products, ensuring that ethical and sustainable standards are met throughout the production process. Consumers are also becoming more conscious of how their beauty and personal care products impact the environment. Choosing castor oil products with certifications such as Fair Trade, Organic, and Rainforest Alliance can help reduce the overall environmental impact while supporting fair labor practices.

The production of castor oil provides livelihoods to thousands of smallholder farmers in rural areas. Social responsibility in castor oil production involves ensuring that these farmers and their communities benefit from the global demand. Companies can play a key role by investing in the communities where castor beans are grown, helping to improve infrastructure, healthcare, and education. Ethical brands often work closely with local farmers, providing training on sustainable farming techniques and ensuring that they are compensated fairly for their crops. By encouraging practices that benefit local economies and protect the environment, the castor oil industry can serve as a model for socially responsible sourcing in the beauty, pharmaceutical, and biofuel sectors.

Chapter Fourteen

Quality Assurance: Selecting the Best Castor Oil

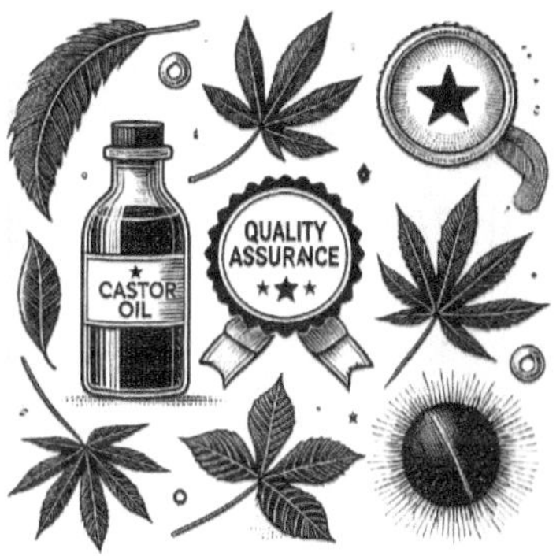

When choosing castor oil for personal or medicinal use, it's essential to understand the factors that determine its quality. With the growing popularity of castor oil across various industries, there are numerous products available on the market. However, not all castor oils are created equal, and selecting a high-quality product can make a significant difference in its effectiveness. This section covers the key factors to consider when choosing castor oil, how to recognize high-quality products, and tips on avoiding low-quality options.

Factors Determining Quality

The quality of castor oil is determined by several factors, including how it's processed, its purity, and the conditions under which the castor beans were grown. High-quality castor oil is usually cold-pressed, which means the oil is extracted from the beans without using heat or chemicals. This method preserves the oil's natural properties, including its ricinoleic acid content, which is responsible for many of its beneficial effects. Cold-pressed oils tend to retain more nutrients compared to those produced through heat extraction, which can degrade the oil's quality. Organic certification is also a crucial factor. Organic castor oil is made from castor beans that are grown without synthetic pesticides or fertilizers, making it a safer and more environmentally friendly choice.

Recognizing High-Quality Products

High-quality castor oil should have a pale yellow color and a thick, viscous consistency. It should be free from impurities, chemicals, or additives. When purchasing castor oil, look for labels that mention "cold-pressed" or "hexane-free," as these indicate a pure extraction process. Hexane is a chemical solvent sometimes used in oil extraction, and while it speeds up production, it can leave trace chemicals in the final product. Organic certifications from reputable organizations, such as USDA Organic or Soil Association, further assure that the oil meets high standards for purity and safety. Additionally, high-quality castor oil will have a mild, neutral scent. If the oil smells rancid or off, it could be a sign of poor processing or improper storage.

Avoiding Low-Quality Options

Low-quality castor oil is often processed with heat or chemicals, which can degrade its beneficial properties. Oils that are overly refined or contain synthetic additives should be avoided, as they may not offer the same therapeutic effects. Dark or cloudy oils may indicate impurities or the presence of contaminants, and these should be avoided. Products that don't clearly label their extraction methods or list the ingredients can also be suspect. It's essential to read reviews and research brands before purchasing to ensure you're not buying a subpar product that has been diluted or mixed with other oils.

Reputable Brands and Sources

Choosing a reputable brand can save you from the guesswork of determining quality. Brands that focus on organic, cold-pressed castor oil are often more reliable. Popular and reputable brands like **Heritage Store**, **Sky Organics**, and **Now Solutions** are known for providing high-quality, organic, cold-pressed castor oils. These brands adhere to ethical sourcing and sustainability standards, ensuring you get a product that is both effective and responsibly produced. Purchasing castor oil from trusted health stores, certified online retailers, or directly from the brand's website can help ensure you're getting an authentic product.

By considering factors like the production method, purity, and the reputation of the brand, you can select the best castor oil for your needs, ensuring both effectiveness and ethical sourcing. Let me know if you'd like more details on any of these aspects!

Conclusion

As we reflect on the journey through castor oil's many uses, it becomes clear that this humble oil plays a far more significant role than most people might expect. Whether you're here to improve your beauty regimen, boost your overall wellness, or explore sustainable alternatives for everyday products, castor oil offers a wealth of possibilities. We've dived deep into its applications, ranging from skincare and hair care to health remedies and ethical production practices. At its core, this book champions the idea of reconnecting with nature's power—utilizing simple, natural solutions that have stood the test of time.

The central message that shines through is that castor oil represents not just a product but a philosophy. Its use stretches back through centuries of human history, touching various cultures and civilizations. Ancient Egyptians, Ayurvedic practitioners, and traditional healers have all valued its remarkable properties, and today, we continue to unlock new benefits through modern science. In doing so, castor oil serves as a reminder that sometimes the most effective remedies come not from a lab, but from the earth. In a world dominated by synthetic solutions and fast-paced lifestyles, castor oil beckons us to slow down and trust in nature's inherent wisdom.

The significance of ethical sourcing has also been a recurring theme throughout this book. In an era of growing environmental awareness, it's crucial that we consider the impact of our choices not only on our bodies but on the planet. By choosing products that are organically grown, sustainably sourced, and fairly traded, we help foster a world where both people and the environment are respected. Castor oil's role in sustainable farming practices and its potential to reduce our reliance on chemical-laden products demonstrate its contribution to a more responsible, eco-conscious lifestyle. The journey to finding sustainable, natural solutions doesn't have to be complex—it can start with simple products like castor oil.

Looking back, it's easy to see why castor oil continues to grow in popularity. It offers a combination of natural efficacy and simplicity that appeals to a wide range of users. Whether it's the anti-inflammatory properties that help soothe sore muscles or the hydrating qualities that leave skin and hair healthier, castor oil proves itself time and again. From beauty enthusiasts to holistic health practitioners, those who have integrated castor oil into their routines often find it to be a reliable, multi-functional product that meets a variety of needs.

As you reflect on what you've learned, I encourage you to view castor oil not just as another product but as an integral part of a broader commitment to health, beauty, and sustainability. Personalizing your use of castor oil is where its true power lies—whether you're using it to enhance your skin, strengthen your hair, or ease discomfort. Tailor its use to fit your unique needs and lifestyle, and don't be afraid to experiment with it. This is a product that invites creativity. Its versatility means you can adapt it to your personal routine, discovering new ways it can improve your well-being and contribute to a healthier, more sustainable life.

But this journey doesn't end with you alone. One of the most exciting aspects of using natural products like castor oil is joining a community of like-minded individuals who share your commitment to natural wellness. Share your experiences with others, learn from their stories, and inspire those around you to make the shift toward more natural, ethical solutions.

Castor oil is more than just an ingredient—it's a conversation starter, a tool for building a healthier world, and a symbol of the powerful connection between human beings and the natural world.

Looking forward, the future of health and beauty lies in embracing simplicity, sustainability, and nature's proven remedies. As more people return to natural products and holistic solutions, castor oil will continue to play a vital role in shaping a more conscious, health-focused culture. This book is just the beginning of your journey with castor oil. As you move forward, stay curious, keep experimenting, and remember that the answers to many of life's challenges are often rooted in nature. Castor oil serves as a testament to the lasting impact of natural remedies, and with continued exploration, there's no limit to what you can discover and achieve.

Keeping the Game Alive

Now that you have everything you need to unlock radiant skin, thicker hair, and natural detoxification, it's time to pass on your newfound knowledge and show other readers where they can find the same benefits.

Simply by leaving your honest opinion of this book on Amazon, you'll show other learners where they can find the information they're looking for and pass their passion for health and wellness forward.

Thank you for your help. The knowledge about peptides is kept alive when we pass on our knowledge – and you're helping us to do just that.

Simply scan the QR code below to leave your review:

Your feedback makes a huge difference and helps others achieve their health goals just like you did. Thank you for being a part of this journey.

References

Int J Naturopath Med

Evidence for the Topical Application of castor Oil – International Journal of Naturopathic Medicine. (2012, March 13).

Skin Type Solutions

Skin Type Solutions. (2024, February 3). *The science of castor oil in skin care products.*

Pretty farm girl

Keel, J. (2024, July 29). *Why castor oil deserves a place in your natural beauty routine.* Pretty Farm Girl. https://prettyfarmgirl.com/blogs/educational/why-castor-oil-deserves-a-place-in-your-natural-beauty-routine

Skin Type Solutions

Skin Type Solutions. (2024b, February 3). *The science of castor oil in skin care products.* https://skintypesolutions.com/blogs/skincare/the-science-of-castor-oil-in-skin-care-products

My Blog

Da Silva, C. (2024, March 10). What Does Castor Oil Do for Skin - CastorOilGuru: Unlock Nature's Secret to Wellness. *My Blog.* https://castoroilguru.com/what-does-castor-oil-do-for-skin/

Thank You for Reading

If you enjoyed this collection, you might also find value in other books by Optilife Publishing. Each title is crafted to help you unlock new levels of health and vitality through natural remedies and cutting-edge insights.

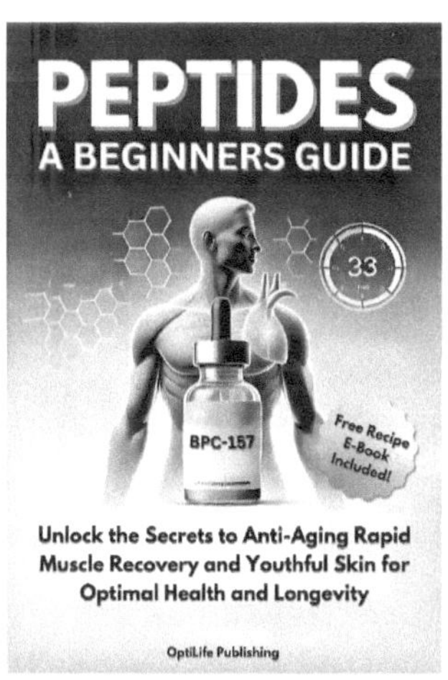

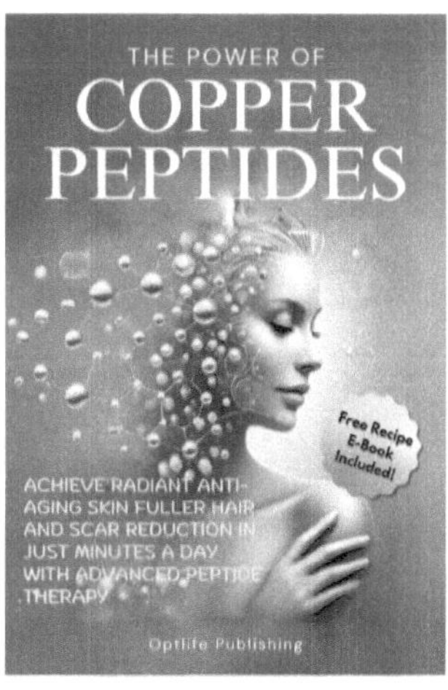

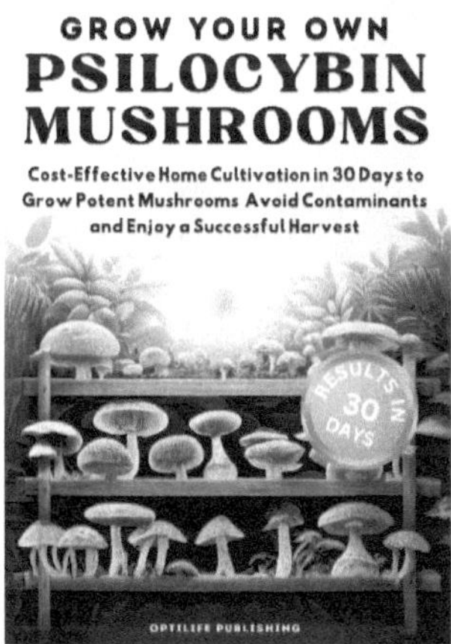

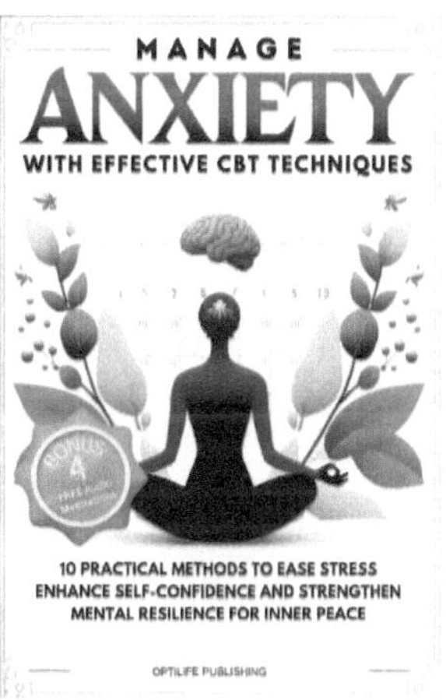

available at 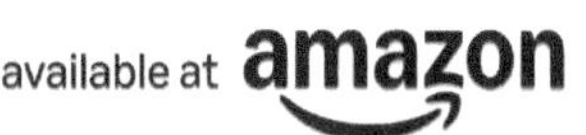

9 798345 082362